Accept that you are imperfect

Writing by

JADE GRANTHAM &
SARAH MICHELLE

Produced by Softwood Books, Suffolk, UK

Published by: Grantham Publishing

This story is based on true events. The names of real people have been changed to protect their privacy.

First Edition
Paperback ISBN: 978-1-3999-7480-6

www.softwoodbooks.com

To my younger self, and to anyone currently going through their own *fight*... one day at a time x

CONTENTS

FOREWORD
AND TRIGGER WARNING

Dear reader,

The words on these pages will not provide the cure for bulimia nor provide the answer for the perfect recovery – how can it, if my own story is still being written? Instead, I want to share the truth behind my journey with bulimia and what I've come to understand caused it. This is where things get tricky. Throughout my story you will read about the struggles I faced both internally and externally. You will read the words I feared saying for so long. Some of these words will describe the acts of bingeing and purging in vivid detail. Others will focus on my inner turmoil. All are carefully considered, not for sensationalism or to create drama worth reading about, instead it is about authenticity, telling the truth that hurts and opening up to the extent that others might be able to identify with what was, and in some ways will always be, my reality.

There is so much focus on 'recovery', however for me, that means it's too late. I believe more needs to be done about prevention so that the point of recovery never needs to be reached. I believe that if we spend more time trying to have the right conversations and uncover what causes so many millions to suffer in the first place, then maybe we can make a bigger impact, and prevent the suffering altogether.

I want to help others see that there is so much more to life than the rules we tell ourselves we must follow, at such a young age. Rules that are informed and compounded by the mass media, fed by small comments that might have been uttered by well-meaning others, or that photo that was taken from the wrong angle. I want this for others, because I still wish I understood the complexity of what I was doing to my body and to myself at the time I was doing it. But, perhaps above all, I wish I had a safer outlet available to me, to understand and admit that I was suffering, which would have prevented years of pain and distress, all of which was self-inflicted because of the mental illness that is bulimia.

Bulimia (Bulimia Nervosa) is a medically diagnosable illness. It is an eating disorder and mental health condition, one of a number that also includes Anorexia Nervosa (food/calorie limiting) and Orthorexia (excessive exercising). Practically speaking, those who have bulimia have periods where they eat a lot of food in a short amount of time, which is called binge-eating, or bingeing. This is often in an out-of-control way where the person doing it feels driven to continue to fill their body with food. Following this overeating, sufferers then cause themselves to be sick, use laxatives designed to quickly release bowels, or engage in excessive exercise to shed any perceived weight gained from bingeing. These behaviours are known as purging and, like bingeing, are usually secretive behaviours and so those suffering are hard to detect, especially in the early days while habits are developing.

It is widely accepted that people who do this, do so primarily as a means of control and/or emotional suppression and release, which is often centred on body weight and image. People can fear putting on weight and can be overly critical of their shape, weight, and body in general. They can also suffer mood swings and often find themselves feeling intense suffering and anxiety, unable to handle everyday situations.

Anyone can become bulimic, but it is more common in young people and teenagers. My suffering started at the age of twelve, before anybody who knew me would have thought I'd be susceptible to the pressures of puberty and the outside world. That's why I believe widespread education and intervention is needed at a young age, before the issues become too big to overcome.

On the cusp of puberty, children are awash with new and ever-changing hormones that run rampant, causing chaos in terms of their wellbeing. Their thoughts and emotions can become confusing and even distressing. At this age, children are trapped in between two worlds, one where the excitement of the perceived freedom of adulthood is intoxicatingly attractive, and at the same time full of their worst fears. One where the bubble-wrapped safety net of family is comfortingly close, and at the same time excruciatingly so.

It's at this time that lots of children seek to gain control over an aspect of their lives, as they hurtle through their tumultuous teen days. Unsurprisingly, this too often manifests in unhealthy habits, and while a little rebellion is a widely accepted right-of-passage in most childhood journeys, the scales are far too easily tipped in our contemporary societies.

The London Centre for Eating Disorders and Body Image Issues have found that the number of children and young people admitted to hospital with eating disorders has increased by 35% in the last year, alone. The Centre explains, 'Almost 10,000 children and young people started NHS eating disorder treatment between April and December 2021– an increase of a quarter compared to the same period the previous year'. However, this figure does not include those young people who entered private treatment, or those who like me, sought no treatment at all, meaning the overall figures, if recorded, would be significantly higher.

In 2005, when I first made myself sick, Our World in Data, suggest 0.05% of the global population between the ages of 5 and 14 were suffering an eating disorder.

The pressures I faced are clearly still there and while I have noticed the conversation around eating disorders expand and move along in a more open and honest manner, the rise in these statistics alarms me and motivates me to act.

Now, with my story, I hope to connect the millions of people who have experienced something similar and encourage them to stop avoiding the help that is being offered.

I want others to know that 'this' doesn't have to be their life.

My ultimate goal is to help provide a deeper understanding as to what is beneath the surface of bulimia so that those suffering, and those close to people who are suffering, can speak out and recover.

Chapter One

TWELVE

Can you remember when you were twelve? What things did you like? Dislike? What kind of child were you?

I was the twelve year-old that was sporty, popular, and confident; on the surface at least.

I was also twelve the first time I forcefully made myself sick after I had eaten a big meal.

I was twelve when I googled 'thinspo' websites and idealised the frighteningly skinny women on the screen.

I was twelve when I lost 8 kg in a matter of weeks.

I was twelve when I lied to everyone around me and pretended I was fine, so that no one would ask questions.

I was twelve when I used to take a shower after every meal, so that I could go to bed empty.

I was twelve when I would come home from school and binge on cereal and then go for a run, so that I could be sick, away from my bathroom in case my mum could smell it.

I was twelve when I had scabs on my knuckles from where my teeth caught the tops of my hands, when I stuck my fingers down my throat.

I was twelve when I felt unhappy with my appearance and punished myself for it.

I was twelve when I stopped processing emotions properly and instead, released everything I was feeling through a vicious cycle of binge and purge.

I was twelve when I used to waste money on binge foods, and hours on getting rid of the food I had just consumed.

I was twelve when no matter how many people could see I was in pain and were actively wanting to help, I pushed them away so that I was isolated and alone.

I was twelve when I became bulimic, something I still deal with every day and while it broke me and caused me an insurmountable amount of pain, the experience I went through, is not something I will ever forget and not something I ever intend to.

Every day I put a small piece of myself back together, and work hard to stay recovered, but I wouldn't change any of it because it has made me the person I am today: Someone I am proud of, someone who appreciates their body for everything it is capable of. Someone who can fully feel and process each emotion, as it comes and reflectively take the time to understand why. Avoidance is never the answer, and I am grateful to finally believe that.

My story begins, unusually, in Malaysia. I was born to expat parents in a suburb, just outside of Kuala Lumpur city centre, where jungle and modern cityscape coexist in harmony. Malaysia is a Southeast Asian country known for its diverse culture, rich history, and stunning natural beauty. My parents were British and while we weren't the only expats in the area, we were certainly in a minority there among the locals and other nationalities.

On the outside, my childhood in Malaysia was so full of picture-perfect experiences – I couldn't wish to have had better! But sadly, this is something I was only able to appreciate and reflect fondly on at a later stage in my life.

At the time, my family and I were happy and comfortable belonging to a society that committed to and celebrated cultural diversity, but, even as a young child, I felt subtle differences between what my eyes saw as the natural beauty of the locals and what I saw when I looked in the mirror at myself.

Similarly, I couldn't shake my self-comparisons with my brother, who at three years older than me seemed to thrive – I felt forever in his shadow. Everything I did, just wouldn't measure up, or at least that's how I felt, back then. In reality, this wasn't the case at all, he was simply older, going through the life stages ahead of me and so just achieving things first.

Growing up, I was *'average sized'*, not really under or overweight by western standards (although not a measure I agree with, I was considered healthy according to the widely used Body Mass Index). In comparing my size, I never made the connection that there were cultural influences that undoubtedly impacted body types, that it might have been my genetic makeup that made my body look different to the ones I coveted and, in reality, prevented me from ever being like them. After all, I was only twelve and this concept was beyond my comprehension and compounded by the lack of awareness of the adults around me. Stanfield et al, (2012), suggest differences in body type compositions between South Asian infants and white Europeans are evident from early infancy and have more to do with genetics, rather than diet, but how can a child make sense of all that?

As my body continued to grow, my worries grew too, at an alarming rate. I quickly became used to obsessively comparing myself to others and to always coming up short in doing so. All I saw were effortlessly light, small-framed bodies surrounding me and I just didn't fit. I would go shopping and try on new clothes that would reveal me to be a Medium to Large size, while the majority of the clothes in the shops were X-Small and Small. My hips were much wider, my frame much thicker.

Today I know comparison really is the thief of joy and everybody is unique, everybody is different and that's the beautiful thing about us, but back then, things for me were spiralling out of control!

Food is a central aspect of Malaysian culture where the unique blend of Malay, Indian, and Chinese cuisines and its abundance of street food vendors make it highly affordable, and a sociable activity enjoyed by all. It was also an obvious connection to make with my dissatisfaction of myself – eating equalled growth and the more I grew, the more my differences stood out and the unhappier I became. And so, I went from what appeared to be disinterest (which in actuality was me convincing myself I was not allowed to like the taste of foods because they would be too tempting to consume), to a learned dislike by the age of twelve.

I grew up unaware that my potentially normal, everyday worries, superpowered by teen hormones and misinterpreted as dissatisfaction with my external self, were piling up inside me. How do we recognise that life isn't normal, when it's all we've ever known?

I was not vocalising my angst, (perhaps because I did not realise I could), and by the time I did, it was unfortunately too late. I had formed destructive patterns of thinking and behaviours and was over-comparing everything I did with my brother, and with friends and, of course, I was always coming up short.

Looking back, I think, even if I had realised what my worries were and that they were growing exponentially, I still wouldn't have been able to connect the dots and understand what was happening to me. Instead, I became more and more certain the problem was me and my weight, and the answer was loss; I just wouldn't have entertained anything in between. If I was the problem, then I could fix the problem!

These comparative thoughts quickly turned into self-hatred and my dissatisfaction with my physical self, became stronger and stronger with each passing day, and the physical discomfort I felt was only matched by the critical internal voice constantly telling me something had to change. Suddenly, my obsession with weight loss gave me a focus, a goal and a solution – I became even more competitive, allowing my addictive personality to cross a new line and, unbeknownst to me, this one would be hell to return from ...

Innocently, as all twelve-year-olds are, I was just making my way through life, learning at school, making friends, and getting good at sports. I grew in popularity because I played everything at school; netball, football, and swimming – here my competitive nature was celebrated and even coveted by my peers. But, despite my love of sports, using the changing rooms often became another source of distress for me. Of course, I was comparing, as usual, and enduring the shameful feelings over my own body image. And rather than getting fired up for the sports I'd be changing for, I found myself constantly, quietly staring at everyone's slimmer frames, especially during swimming practice, by the pool.

As my body grew, life did what it does and threw new obstacles in my way. Somehow, I developed noticeable stretch marks all over my backside. I was just growing, but night after night, sleep was increasingly hard to come by as I hysterically cried over these marks. For me, all of a sudden, my fears had been confirmed and I could actually see a 'result' of me being too big.

The name itself, 'stretch marks', which can happen naturally in puberty, and have nothing to do with being overweight, haunted me. My mum recognised my distress (bless her) and tried with all the home remedies she could think of to help me, including exfoliating. Eventually the stretch marks faded, as they do, but by that time, I had already made myself thinner.

I always had such a negative perception of things like stretch marks and cellulite. I felt strongly that it was my fault and I had failed because I had it, despite it being a very natural phenomenon happening to my body (nobody ever discussed this in terms of growing up!) All I knew was that I had to be better than that. I couldn't have marks because they would make me ugly. There was absolutely no normalising it, only fixing or removing it, as if it is a problem. Now, at nearly thirty years old, I know it's natural, it's healthy and thankfully, it is being normalised more with unfiltered 'real' images of people online, however back then only photoshop and models were on show. Imagine trying to explain to a child that it was not real, when that is all they saw.

At home, normal to houses in Asia, every bedroom had its own bathroom, a feature which became a very convenient tool to mask my behaviour in the early days. *I wonder if I had grown up in the UK, where there were often only shared bathrooms, whether my story would be very different?*

When and how much I ate, was (like most children), controlled by my parents, who loved food (as did my brother). Our house was always full of very healthy, balanced food. I'm very aware that while growing up like this, I was luckier than a lot of children, but I couldn't see or understand that, and it all became a burden for me. Every time my parents called upstairs to say 'dinner was ready' my heart sank.

Early on in my life, my parents observed my behaviour around food was different from theirs. My attitude would range from nonchalant to perceived disgust and so my dad, for whom cooking was a passion, would go above and beyond making special alternatives to the main family meal, just to encourage me. It must've been so hard to understand having one child so eager to eat everything in sight, experiment with new tastes and textures and find obvious pleasure in doing so, and then to have me! It must have been frustrating too, to never be able to satisfy their daughter in terms of food, especially when they'd go to such lengths to include me in family meals.

Now I understand my dad was trying to be accommodating and offer me support through the act of making different meals he thought I'd enjoy, and it was his way of caring. Back then, I just saw it as me being made to feel more difficult and a cause of conflict; he was preventing me from my goal and another contributor to my self-hatred.

On top of this, my internal fears were being compounded by seemingly innocent external influences. From an early age, I had noticed that some of the adults around me would sort of diet from time to time. They would restrict their food intake (especially carbs) when they felt unhappy with their own appearance which was normally deemed to be a result of weight gain or overindulging. This was despite my parents not being overweight in the slightest, no one in our life was really, which made it even harder for me to understand why I fantasised about being unhealthily underweight.

And, even in the age before social media really took off, it was impossible not to notice the fads and diets touted as the 'next best thing' for the masses to achieve their weight loss goals. Magazine pages, film and TV ads, websites, and then old-fashioned word-of-mouth spread these messages far and wide to millions of people around the world. Weight loss and fitness tools started to appear outside of health food shops and took their place on everyday shop shelves where they slipped into the subconscious minds of children trying to work out just how the world worked.

Of course, my impressionable young mind took it all in. All I saw was this 'type A' person with the perfect body, which, (mixed in with my obsessive nature), became a dangerous cocktail that would drive me to find ways to make a much bigger impact on my size. I became obsessive about cutting out my fear foods, the 'bad' foods, which were of course carbs like pasta, rice, and bread. My naivety is almost hilarious to me now; I didn't even know that fruit was a carbohydrate! In fact, I didn't know anything of substance as to the macro and micronutrients in food and just how they fuelled our bodies. I was simply a little girl who made up a rule and then stuck by it for over ten years. I was twenty-seven years old the first time I ate a pizza, without guilt, shame, or a sense of dread. Where did I learn that pizza was bad? From the same sources that purported 'if you want to lose weight you don't eat pasta!'

One of the early tactics I did to reduce the amount of food I'd have to eat, was to ask if I could be vegetarian. This happened around the age of nine. My mum vetoed the idea quickly, (I didn't eat a lot of vegetables, so she feared for my health and thankfully put her foot down). So as a compromise, I still ate seafood on occasion. My motivations were not to do with ethical and moral beliefs surrounding animals or because my body did not agree with eating meat, it was all towards that one elusive goal.

It was around this time I started to lie with ease to hide the scary internal truth. A skill I would rely on and perfect over the years. Of course, if anyone asked, it was all about the welfare of animals. But I'd quickly realised that, when looking at a menu, I had less choice and temptation staring me in the face, and from what I could falsely see online, vegetarians were thinner!

Within three short years, I went from restricting my food intake to look better, as much as a child possibly could (without raising all-out-alarm), to blaming all my anxieties and problems on the way I looked, which was compounded as I scoured the internet for inspiration and solutions to achieve that size zero look, that I felt so far away from: I was silently spiralling.

Inside, I felt like I was running out of options to fix my issues before I drowned in them and my young mind (unbeknownst to anyone else, including me) had begun making unhelpful, and even dangerous connections in my subconscious. Thin people were obviously happier and If I was thin, I would be happy and I would be perfect. All I needed was a way.

Then, on a very normal day at primary school, during a science class, we were taught about the basics of food and nutrition, and this is where I first learned about eating disorders. I was fascinated by the subject, and, through blinkered vision, I felt like I had finally been spoken to and had found a solution. I did not listen to the side effects or impact of these disorders, all I heard, loudly and clearly as if calling directly to my subconscious mind, was that they were a quick method of weight loss.

Finally (with my new solution), I could live a normal life, for all intents and purposes, and even let myself enjoy some things and none of it would matter. I could prevent weight gain, and release all of my built-up anxiety in one visit to the bathroom.

To my twelve-year-old self it was very black and white. Food in vs food out; it was my only concern and here was an easy fix. In reality, the release of food after each meal also meant a release of my emotional state, which, back then, was overbearing. It became almost like a game.

I vividly remember the first time I tried to make myself sick. I was on holiday with my family in Spain where I put on a brave face. The trouble was that every time I put on my bikini, or even everyday clothes, I felt that deep angst and frustration when I looked in the mirror. My body image was all consuming and the negative voice in my head was growing louder and louder, seemingly every day.

I couldn't appreciate the beach because all I saw were perfect bikini bodies. They were everywhere I looked (because that's exactly what I chose to see), and I was addicted to looking at their thin, beautiful bodies and associating it with their perfect lives: I couldn't imagine ever feeling that confident, but I so craved it.

Of course, there must have been very different body types filling those beaches; young children, old people, the active and inactive, those from very different cultures, but they just didn't exist in my vision. I'm also very aware now, that there's a good chance that I wasn't alone sitting there, oblivious to my family and the natural beauty around me, coveting what I didn't have.

At this point, I'd already decided what beauty was (or rather, I'd fallen into the trap of believing I knew what beauty was), from the media parading around on my screen and on page, after page, after page on the internet. Beauty (which in my head already equalled happiness), was 0% body fat and given that all the major fashion houses and designer brands employed size zero models to sell their clothes, it's easy to see how I had fallen into that trap and subscribed to that belief. Don't get me wrong, no one ever said out loud to me that I didn't fit this ideal, they did not need to, the parades of perfect bodies decorating the social media and tabloid pages did all the talking for them. Even today, I know that millions of women crave that 'ideal' body type because of those pictures on the pages.

The pursuit of that 'perfect' shape fuelled my addictive personality and became, not surprisingly, an all-consuming set of thought patterns that distracted me from my holiday and uninterrupted quality time with my family. There was no respite, even away from the beach where my size 4 cousin drew my envious gaze, appearing to effortlessly fit that beautiful stereotype I so desired: I was jealous. At no point did I think we had different genetics, we were different body shapes, and even ages. I just compared my size directly to hers and knew I was bigger and therefore less than.

You can see where this is going, right? Even if I had told anyone how I was feeling, or of my destructive thought patterns, I would not have listened to their replies. For a twelve-year-old, I was stubborn and determined that I knew best. I was also at a point of desperation, where no measure seemed too extreme in the pursuit of what I believed was the answer to unlocking my happiness. The way I (thought I) saw it, my body and I were disconnected. I couldn't see that my body was able, that it was healthy and that it needed to be looked after, I just wanted, no needed it to be better.

So, at a time that is meant to bring families closer together, instead I became more disconnected. We'd been out for a family meal in a typical Spanish restaurant and afterwards, though my family wasn't that far away, in my head, I felt completely alone.

I had overeaten at dinner, and I felt like I had failed, I had let myself down and I couldn't stand the feeling of fullness. It was at that moment that I went into the bathroom of the restaurant, turned the tap on full, took a deep breath and made myself sick for the first time.

Though I did feel some apprehension in not knowing how this would go, being immersed in that moment prevented me from appreciating the potential consequences of my actions on my own future. I couldn't have known the impact it would cause in my relationships with other people, with myself and how it would become a part of my everyday life – even today. That one moment changed everything for me.

In a bathroom, in a restaurant, while on holiday, I did not think, I did not feel, I just turned everything off and I acted. I gingerly pushed my fingers toward the back of my throat and waited for it to hurt, for me to have to push further, be more committed, for it to be harder. But it wasn't. The worst thing of all happened, I found it easy and worse, rewarding. After I had expelled the food, I became flooded with an overwhelming sense of relief that quickly converted to happiness. I felt euphoric!

I now recognise this feeling as coming from setting out to, and having achieved, my goal, but at the time, to my young mind, it reinforced those actions as having been right for me.

I left that bathroom satisfied and externally I was more engaged with my family, more talkative, more at ease Internally, I cradled my secret and felt hopeful that this was the start of my journey toward physical perfection and happiness, and away from all my problems.

I purged once more on that holiday, again finding it far too easy and more than a little satisfying. I congratulated myself each time I prevented the food I'd just eaten, being converted into body fat. And I knew I'd continue when I got home, in fact, I knew I'd look harder, read more, and find other ways to help me shrink in size. What I didn't know was that however easy it had been for me to start; it would be a hundred times harder for me to stop.

It wasn't until I was twenty, over eight years later, that I realised what I was doing everyday – the hours, the money, the emotional, mental, and physical damage to myself – was wrong and that I needed help. I was sick, every day, often several times a day for eight years, which is over **2900** days. When converted into time spent in the bathroom with my fingers covered in vomit, eyes streaming, and stomach acid burning my oesophagus, it equates to over **4000** hours. I find it hard to comprehend the amount of time I wasted in the pursuit of being perfect, a goal that I was never going to achieve, because it does not exist. But, of course, I didn't know that then.

I've been asked, if I had the chance to go back to the first time I made myself sick and not do so, would it have prevented me from the years and years of suffering that followed? Knowing me, it wouldn't have made a difference, I would have found a way, if not that day, then another day and I would have achieved my goal. It's only now, through the painful journey of it all, that I was able to truly force myself to understand, confront my fears and to accept what happened, making me the strong woman I am today, aware of all my flaws and able to manage them to truly live a fulfilling and happy life.

Now, I accept that I am imperfect.

Chapter Two

THIRTEEN

Psychological studies have indicated that it takes an average of sixty-sixdays to form a habit, (Lally 2009). When it comes to food habits, this can be even quicker, for example, the NHS suggest that for babies to accept new tastes and textures, it takes an average of ten tries or more.

I don't know the exact amount of binge-purge cycles it took for me to form my habit, but I do know the many rules I'd convinced myself I had to follow, quickly became an all-consuming aspect of my life. And my competitive, disciplined nature meant that I was always pushing myself, in whatever I did, to be better.

I always associated my bulimia with my weight, I now know that was only one of the symptoms. When I became overwhelmed, I purged. When I felt anxious, I purged. Whenever I felt under any sort of external or internal pressure, I would purge. And it became addictive, the sense of euphoria and relief I'd feel in the moments following a purge became my reward, and on top of that, I enjoyed having my secret. I felt powerful and it was addictive.

I stopped being able to differentiate between my emotions. Whatever I felt, I just waited for the next mealtime to get that sense of release. Any time I was uncomfortable, physically or emotionally, I knew what I needed to do.

Achieving things can become a bit of an addiction too. It feels good to accomplish the goals we set for ourselves, and we are ultimately rewarded with a sense of control over our lives, (though we might not always recognise it) and so we are more easily convinced to repeat the behaviours that won the sense of achievement, in the future. I created patterns and routines that made me feel good on the surface. For example, as a family, we'd always sit and watch TV together after our evening meal. I planned to use this time to be sick in my shower, knowing my family would be distracted enough not to ask too many questions and when this plan worked, it felt good. The heightened stress of not knowing if I would be able to get away with it that night, and then the relief once it was all done. I'd succeeded and I liked that feeling, so of course I'd pursue it again and again. I am someone that even to this day, loves routine! Sure, I would get push back from my parents as to why I was missing out on quality family time, but I would be hostile and say I wanted to be alone!

I didn't know at the time, of course, that I was trying to gain a semblance of control in my life, but now, looking back at my twelve-year-old self, I can see why I would, why anybody at that age would. All I knew was that sense of achievement each time I purged, along with relief, overwhelming relief, and it was better than anything I felt in between those times. At such a young age all I could control in my life was food and, on the surface, it did the trick.

I carried on with the facade of everything being just fine; externally I was thriving, and I felt happier, I was getting thinner. And at first, I thought I was hiding my truth well. I learned quickly what to avoid eating based on food that was hard to purge and nothing else. I avoided foods like rice because I would be in the bathroom or shower for an extra thirty minutes, trying to get every grain out. I wouldn't stop until I knew there was nothing left. I was obsessive and even though what remained was probably equal to one calorie, I had to be completely empty.

Still, I went to school each day just like anybody else. Then I'd come home, close the door to the outside world and binge on unhealthy snacks, like cereal, before the inevitable purging followed, disguised by going to my room and doing homework with loud music on.

When I wasn't at school, in addition to my food intake rules, I'd go out for runs, often being sick on these runs to make it easier to hide. I'd also make sure I'd complete at least 100 sit-ups a day, which left bruises down my spine, not that it mattered to me. We had weighing scales at home and, of course, I made use of them, checking my weight every morning and after every purge, making sure it never went up – seeing a 0.1kg increase would make me hysterical.

When I wasn't concentrating on weight loss, I became comfortable spending more time in my head, above all other places, finding peace in privacy alone. I had a big secret, and it was all mine. My greatest confidant and source of support was me, but I was also my worst enemy, ignoring the signs that things weren't going so well and convincing myself I must continue to follow the rules I'd set for myself around food.

As my rules and actions started to take their toll on my body, I retreated further inward and convinced myself there was no one that would understand the way I felt and what I needed to do. My primary school was small, and my outer circle of friends was naturally shrinking as we neared the end of that period of our lives, no one there noticed that I was shrinking too. I'd be moving onto boarding school eventually, following in my brother's footsteps, but I didn't spend much time thinking about it as more of my waking hours focused on achieving my weight goals.

Around this time, a close friend of mine was discovered to have an eating disorder. Her appearance dramatically changed in a very short space of time and there was lots of fuss made about how skinny she'd become. I now know most of that fuss would have been 'alarm', but it seemed to me that everyone had just become aware of her weight loss, not the dangerous side effects. I saw a girl that looked like I wanted to look, and I saw that her methods had worked and now she had everybody trying to figure out how to solve her problems. This didn't make me more aware of the dangerous effects of my behaviours. Instead, my perception was so warped that I was jealous. I knew I had to try harder.

It wasn't long before the physical effects were obvious, my skin started to suffer, drying out and breaking out regularly on my face. I also had scabs forming on my skin, where my teeth clashed with my knuckles as I forced them down my throat. My hip bones protruding, bruises on my spine. I could sense the worry start to grow around me, but *I must not get caught*, I thought to myself, *I don't want to stop, and no one can force me to.*

At the time, I thought I was happily locked up in my head with my feelings and actions all reinforced by my bulimia. The illness assured me I was OK, applauded my determination, and stayed with me through it all. She kept the world at arm's length, forming an almost impenetrable wall between me and anyone who dared judge, criticise, or even advise against my way of thinking.

Now I know better. I know things were out of control for me and what I needed, what I really needed, I couldn't understand, let alone vocalise. And if I couldn't understand it myself, no one else was even going to get close. I thought I wanted the world to look away and let me get on with what I knew would make my life better, but now I'm not so sure I did. Now, I am sure things would've been better if the world hadn't.

Despite family and school friends starting to notice and worry about me (I'd gone from around 60 kg to 44 kg), the reactions were not all negative. Some girls praised me for my new look, which acted as positive reinforcement. I think, deep down, (despite the compliments), I knew what I was doing was harmful and so it was easy to think I would be judged harshly, looked down upon, thoughtless of, be disappointed in ... and I wasn't strong enough to face that, so I hid more, spoke less, and became even more focused on my body image. I never gave anyone the chance to help me, because at the time I was in total denial to myself.

In reliving that period of my life, I would do anything to be able to 'get through' to my thirteenyear-old self and just tell her it's OK to be afraid, it's OK to not understand, and it's OK to show those close to you your vulnerabilities and pain.

I was lucky, always being so close to my parents and enjoying a beautiful relationship, but I don't recall them ever willingly showing me their own emotional vulnerabilities. I remember they always appeared so kept together; they were so strong, and I thought I had to be like that! Of course, as parents, most think that's how you should act in front of your children, to not to show any weakness, conflict, or emotional distress because it is widely accepted that it's important for children to sense the adults around them are in control, that they know what's what and that they have your back. But if this is the reality, how do children learn that it's OK to be afraid, to ask for help, to cry; how do children accept that it's OK to not know the answer?

Despite their appearance to me, I can't imagine what my parents must've been going through at the time. I do know now that they were scared of what was potentially happening to me and, at times, frustrated by my refusal to talk, or listen, and I can fully appreciate why. I reasoned that they couldn't possibly understand, so there was no point in me trying to talk to them and I really didn't want them to think any less of me, so avoidance – hiding away – was the best option. And pushing them away was easier than letting them in and having them forcing me to stop.

Mum, especially, tried to talk to me about things on so many occasions, but my walls stood strong. Being a nurse, she had recognised the smell of vomit emanating from my bathroom; my scented candles were no disguise when it came to her. She'd try to have nice, non-threatening conversations with me about my health, but I'd hide behind that wall and keep quiet. Each time she asked, I became more hostile in my response. I was scared. I wanted everyone to leave me alone.

At one point, my mum insisted on weighing me weekly, on Sundays, at home. It was awkward for both of us, I'd feel threatened and get angry at the littlest things and she'd try to gently probe and question me with no success. In response, I started going out for more runs to avoid the scrutiny and I'd be sick while out, where I knew there'd be no one waiting to catch me.

I would binge in secret, bowl after bowl of cereal or whatever I could get my hands on in the fridge and cupboards. I'd eat to the point I could hardly move and then I'd put on my running gear, while avoiding my reflection in the mirror, as I was extremely bloated. I would run, get around the corner and out of sight and stick my fingers down my throat. I'd be careful to avoid dog walkers and cars driving by, so they couldn't see my eyes watering from the retching and my fingers covered in chunks of food and saliva. Then I would come home, run again to the shower to wash away any evidence, and then for a couple of hours, a small semblance of peace – I could face the world again. Only for a couple of hours though, then, of course, I would do it all again.

One evening, we went out as a family for a Chinese meal. For a while now, when I'd gone out with friends, I'd taken to asking to be picked up last, delaying it for as long as I could, just so I'd have the time to be sick before I got in the car to go home. This time, with my family already aware of an issue, there'd be nowhere to go ...

That day, I was already moody and shut down because Mum had already been carefully probing before we left the house, probably trying her best to avoid the inevitable conflict that peppered family mealtimes with me. I'd already had the internal argument over whether to eat less and not have to hide being sick, (but put up with the disappointment and concerned comments over my disinterest in the meal) or eat loads and find the time and space to throw it back up again after. As always, the attention I knew I'd draw from my lack of eating horrified me and so I chose to eat and get to the bathroom as soon as I could.

Unfortunately, the lesser of the two evils (as I saw it), still drew attention to me and made my dad snap sternly, *'What is wrong with you?'* as we sat together at the table. What does he mean? How could he understand? I became hysterical, forcibly pushing my parents away for fear that they would make me stop, and I didn't want that, even though it was causing me so much pain; I had not achieved my goal yet and I was not ready. I needed to continue, I needed to keep forcibly making myself sick after every meal.

My parents were beside themselves as my problem had become so visible. They looked at their thin-haired, gaunt, emotionally unstable thirteen-year-old shell of a daughter, who kept telling them she was *fine,* and I can only imagine how helpless they felt. By this point, I was far too deep into my battle to see things from any other perspective, I did not care if they were upset, or suffering, I was hurting more and so I did the only thing I knew how to do – I doubled down and withdrew further into myself.

Around this time, I was at my lowest weight, just 44 kg. I remember getting ready for a friend's birthday party, looking in the mirror, blinded by self-disgust and negativity. It must've been so obvious that I was too thin, but I couldn't see it and certainly never felt it at the time. Now I know, that's the scariness of the illness.

As an adult, it's easy to recognise the overriding state of unhappiness and anxiousness that fed into my behaviours. I can also now recognise that the behaviours themselves exacerbated it all, and I wonder how I ever thought those short moments of relief, that momentary sense of achievement and those seconds-long glances in the mirror ever compensated for it. I guess that's it, I didn't think!

Instead, several times a day, I would switch everything off inside, go into autopilot (so I didn't have to feel anything), and just do what I absolutely knew I needed to do. Back then, I couldn't comprehend what I was doing to my parents, to my juvenile body, to me. I was in so deep, I saw no way of getting out, so I had to keep going.

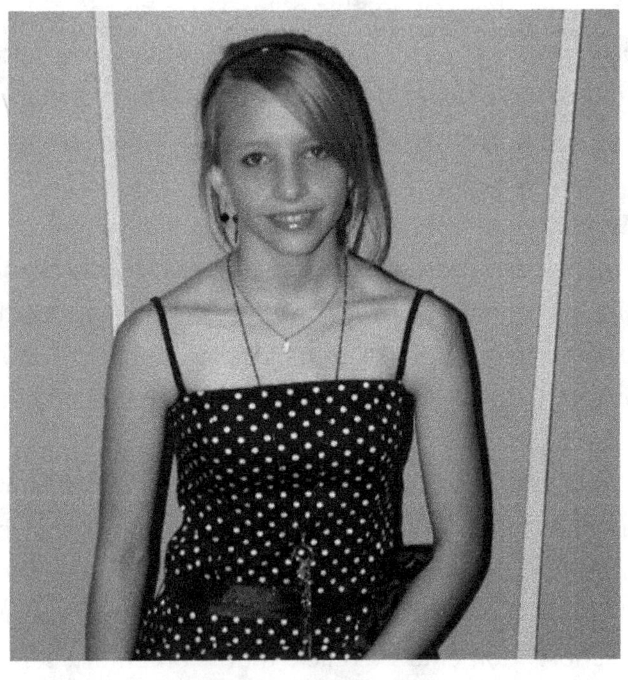

Friends 13th Birthday Party

Chapter Three

FIFTEEN

A study suggests that children become susceptible to social influence, from around the age of twelve, Large et al (2019).

Singapore would be the setting for the next few years of my life, when from the age of fifteen, I attended United World College, an international boarding school there.

I didn't understand at the time, but I've since come to learn that most of the food we eat during a meal is digested in the first ten minutes. I was sick, on average, between thirty and sixty minutes after eating, sometimes longer, so I was keeping most of my calories anyway, working against myself, all that time. Read that again ... after the first ten minutes, all the calories are absorbed which highlights the irrationality of what I did, for eight (plus) years. I had a belief in my head, and no one educated me otherwise. I wonder how many other incorrect and false beliefs people are holding onto and letting them dictate their disordered eating behaviours. I did not need to be told I was damaging my body, my hair, my teeth, all I needed was to be sat down and explained the facts – the truth behind the weight loss method that I had incorrectly fantasised over since that science class in primary school.

It was 2009, and even though the scenery would change, my story would stay the same. I would fall into the same 'self-set' routines that I'd rigidly obeyed at home, as I joined my new classmates for the next stage in my life.

In the run up to my big move, my desperation to leave my turmoil behind had only grown. I was to be the new girl at the boarding house and in my grade at school, but those nerves were easily taken care of. I thought finally, I could be the best version of myself, I could be me (it would be easier for me to get away with bingeing and purging at school, because my parents wouldn't be there to catch me out and make me feel guilty for what I was doing). The only thing I feared was the shared bathrooms, but I knew enough to realise there was no one there who cared about me enough, no one who was close enough to stop me anymore.

And they did not know my secret, and that was enticing. It became a game, and I became very good at my game!

The problem was that my parents had become so worried, that they threatened to not let me go to Singapore, unless I stopped doing what I was doing and became a healthy weight. Of course, I didn't stop then, instead I just became more secretive and managed to maintain more of a healthy weight – they'd have to let me go then!

I found it was so easy to lie to my parents, to friends

and to everyone, because whatever initial guilt I felt in telling the lie, the hold my bulimia had over me was so much more powerful. I would do anything to protect my secrets.

At one point, out of desperation, my mum asked me to go to a local clinic in Malaysia, which terrified me into letting her in a little. It's a very generalised formula; you get admitted, you get weighed, they watch you eat prescribed meals and then, when you reach what in their terms is a healthier weight, you get released. It's shocking to me now, that the root cause was never investigated.

In my experience, there's a huge lack of education in working with children suffering an eating disorder. No professionals tried to support my thinking brain, and nobody tried to undo the dangerous pathways I'd formed in relation to my sense of self and to my place in the world, and so I learnt avoidance – to play the game even better. I simply promised my parents I had stopped, and even put on a little more weight, but in reality, I just delayed my purging until they had gone to bed in the lead up to going to boarding school. Of course, the clinic was a blow to me, but I soon realised the hoops I needed to jump through to get what I wanted. It was only temporary until I could be fully in control again.

Thankfully, I joined my new school at the start of my IGCSE year, full of enthusiasm for the freedom I'd so longed for. I didn't know this at the time, but my mum had spoken with the Houseparent in my dorm about her concerns over my weight and behaviour and they'd agreed that she'd keep a good eye on me and let Mum know if anything seemed wrong, and I do think she tried.

I found fitting in easy enough because externally I was confident, and I was fun to be around. Now I think I was lucky to be in Singapore, one of the world's safest countries, because I dread to think of what *could* have happened, had I been elsewhere, living as I was living. I'd go out clubbing with a fake ID and I'd drink and smoke, stay out all night; I'd get blackout drunk. All the popular kids were doing it, and we were all desperately trying to fit in with one another, following the pack, too afraid of not fitting in to be authentic. *Today my motto is: conformity fits, authenticity doesn't.*

Despite the peer pressure, I know that no one was to blame for my actions, I was one of the main instigators because I loved escaping my own head and my obsessive thoughts about my body. When I was drunk, most of the time, the internal noise was a bit quieter, I felt a bit lighter. Over the years this coping method understandably got worse as my tolerance grew and my chosen methods to quieten everything down reduced in their effectiveness. Out of desperation and in the absence of alternatives, I pushed the boundaries further.

Once I was even arrested for shoplifting. It's another example of how I turned everything off; I was numb to any of the potential consequences. I found it was increasingly easy for me to disconnect myself from my actions and not care. I learned to disengage and simply move through the motions of life. Of course, it was terrifying being caught shoplifting, being arrested and placed in a holding cell, waiting for my disappointed parents to collect me. On the surface, I cried, and I was a little scared, but deep down I didn't really care. I played the victim because I had bigger things to think about – my secret.

Back at school, there were a lot of pressures on me to do well, pressures I now know I created and placed on myself. I was acutely aware that it was costing my parents a lot of money to send me to this school. I also knew that my brother had been doing so well and that called out to the competitive streak in me, so when I wasn't getting into trouble, I was working hard.

Life at boarding school was full-on and, in many ways, I loved it. I carried on playing sports and found a good group of teammates and friends. I even found it easy to purge, as the showers were big and there were heaps of toilets around school that I had access to after hours. Everyone was always busy, and I was pleased to find that no one cared as much as my own parents did in terms of my eating behaviours. I could binge eat after school and at mealtimes and no one ever noticed. And so, it continued to be a part of my daily mealtime routine.

The dinners at the boarding house were buffet-style every night; there was no portion control, it was all in my hands. One evening, I ate so much at dinner that I panicked. I quickly rushed back to one of the toilets that was far away from everyone, it was only a ten-minute walk but that night, it was too far. My body rejected the food on its own and I was sick in a bus stop, in the dark, hiding from everyone. Afterwards, I took a moment to breathe, to look around and check if my secret was still intact. Thankfully, (I thought at the time), no one noticed, and I continued my evening as I did every other.

Interestingly, throughout my boarding years, I ended up causing my mum a lot of angst that I couldn't have foreseen. I would often complain to her about how unhealthy the food was and how hard it was for me to buy my own food because of the cost and the time involved in prepping it. I was projecting my own excuses onto her as to why I continued to be bulimic. My head was in turmoil, and I searched for blame; when I was at home, eating very healthy balanced food, my parents were responsible. At school, the food was to blame. You will see later on in this book, there was always something, as tiny as a reason it may have been, it was always enough to keep my habit alive.

Throughout my boarding years, I managed an active sports life, which fed my competitive nature and helped maintain my weight to a certain degree. Playing sports gave me another, healthier escape from my head, so when I had to, I would compromise and eat for fuel. I loved being a part of a team and feeling that belonging and sense of achievement after games, but sports didn't ever tip the scales; I had my secret and that was separate.

However, I became acutely aware that my body was struggling when my periods abruptly stopped. Fleetingly, I began to question the impact my behaviours might be having on my body, and of the potential consequences of not being able to have a family of my own. But these moments were few and far between, I was young and having a family was no contest for having the peace that I knew would come with achieving my goals. I still believed the answer to most of my problems were in my weight loss, so I numbed myself to those little voices and I continued on. Besides, all the websites and available information I had read said that no periods would be a consequence and potential side effect of my food restrictions and that meant I was doing things correctly.

A key moment for me during my time at school was when I was chosen to play at the 2011 Touch Rugby World Cup in Edinburgh for the Singaporean mixed open team. It was an amazing achievement and still such a fond memory to look back on. However, what clouds those memories (and actually a lot of my family holidays during this time) was the overbearing distress and panic I had in the lead up to the tournament. I would have to wear the spandex material top and shorts on the field, in front of my team members and opposition: I would be seen, and I was not ready.

When there were *special* occasions like these, I would get a bit stricter, I would try to be more controlled causing more mental and physical exhaustion. Even when representing my country in something I loved, I wasn't given a break from my discipline and obsessiveness.

Another stand-out moment was during my final IB exams. Despite managing good grades, consistently throughout all my schooling, when it came to my final exams, the pressure was too much. The more stress I was under, the worse my patterns of bingeing and purging became. Without the routine of classes, I couldn't concentrate, I couldn't be left alone with my own thoughts to try and retain information or revise.

Every time I sat down, opened a book and tried to absorb the information, I wanted to binge and purge and release the stressful feeling. *Just quickly* I would think, or after the next chapter, persuading myself I deserved a snack, a break, a release. I would make notes and notes of information, taking in none of it. Wasting hours of 'revision' when mentally I was elsewhere. I also used to smoke cigarettes a lot, simply because I had seen, in a movie somewhere, that it was an appetite suppressant; it was another escape away from food.

I wasted hours during my study leave, sitting on the bathroom floor with my head shoved down the toilet or on my knees in the shower, leaning over the open drain, desperately trying to mask the smell of the vomit and the noise of the retching. I would make myself sick to the point that I'd become lightheaded. I could hardly stand up; I was dehydrated and tired. So, I would have something to eat ... and the whole cycle would start again.

Thinking back to those moments it amazes me to see the trance I was in, fully escaped and separated from the real world. But it wasn't a shock that I didn't get my grades and did not get into my university of choice. After exams,

I remember being back home in Malaysia with everything crumbling around me because at the time the biggest thing I had needed to achieve, I failed – but inside, I was numb.

I know during this time I was hard to be around, my behaviours seemed selfish and secretive, because they were. I failed to respect boundaries of the people I cared about the most at school and I felt like I was never honest about the real me. They let me in fully, but I never let anyone in. I put up a front and never let them in, which meant when I left school and that life behind me, I was able to easily walk away. I had turned everything off inside me.

I moved back home for the summer and spent hours every day going through my options, trying to get a place at university in the UK through clearing. Eventually, I settled on International Relations at Loughborough University and then I saw a glimmer of hope and I started to countdown the days till I could start over (again). I needed to escape, blaming my externalities for my pain when it should have been obvious – it was me.

Over that summer, I spent more days down, than I did happy, more days shut away in my bedroom, staying up all night and sleeping in for hours all morning, just struggling to cope with the everyday. I was in one of the world's most beautiful countries, surrounded by a family that loved me and all I felt was darkness.

During this period, there was a lot of time for me to think and I soon concluded that enough was enough … Thankfully, my periods had returned (a fact that was celebrated as a sign of my recovery), but it took me a while to feel it, as it meant I was going against my 'goal'. Can you imagine thinking like that? Being glad as a child that you had, through extreme weight loss, caused your body to malfunction.

As I got older and started to think about my future, I had different motivations. I knew I wanted kids (when the time was right) and that created a different motivation in me, a different thought pattern was beginning to emerge. It also showed that despite the behaviours I was undertaking, my weight was normal(ish), and my body was on the right track. It was a different story for my mental state, but I was an expert at disconnecting the two.

I concluded that I could not continue like this. It had been six years of a vicious cycle. I knew at some point I had to stop bingeing and purging because it was the only thing I had a grip on in my life at the moment, everything else was spiralling out of control. There was no denying the effects on my physical health anymore. This would be it; I'd decided.

My bulimia had been consuming to the point where I was purging several times a day, every day. But for what? I was not skinnier; I was not happier. I was just lying to everyone around me, and I did not want to anymore. The smallest of situations I would overreact, over stress, have anxiety attacks – because I could not cope with any of it.

Uni was the fresh start I needed to leave it all behind,

once and for all. I could bury myself in the books and the social scene and more importantly, I was moving to self-catered accommodation where I had 100% control of my food, my meals, and my life. This time would be different; my parents were not there for me to blame, I was no longer at boarding school with canteen-style buffets of unhealthy food and treats where I could have any portion size I wanted to, and there would be no boarding house parents, teachers, or friends' parents to try to control my food. In my head I was doing food shops of vegetables and healthy foods (no carbs of course) and looking the best I ever had. In my head, I was happy. I would finally be an adult, fully in control and no longer suffering ... It would all work out ...

I wish it had.

Chapter Four

EIGHTEEN

Thinspo (thin-inspiration), Pro-Ana (pro-anorexia) and Pro-Mia (pro-bulimia) sites, websites dedicated to providing targeted information and images, tips and tricks with the aim of assisting views to achieve their (under) weight goals. They are supposed to be motivational. The trouble with these sites lies in just how attractive they are to vulnerable people, a lot of whom may have serious questions relating to their health, are seeking to validate their beliefs, or might simply be searching for a community with whom they can share experiences and feel a sense of belonging, especially, when they are hiding so much from those around them in the 'real world'. And while these sites might require the user to explicitly search for them, the same content is often readily available when scrolling through the pages of social media's biggest giants, a place where you are at the mercy of algorithms. In 2021, a whistleblower from Instagram revealed internal research regarding the site's toxic effects, particularly in the rise of eating disorders among children, had been deliberately downplayed by them. And in 2022, despite the platform reinforcing a ban on glorifying eating disorders using human and AI moderation, there were still searchable pro-anorexia hashtags on TikTok.

I moved to university within the town of Loughborough, in 2012 and into self-catered, cluster accommodation on campus, with my own room and shared kitchen and bathroom facilities. With my brother already in his final year at Nottingham university, mum had flown over with me and stayed in between the two of us for a few days, until freshers' week started, when she flew back to Malaysia. I had the usual first-day nerves, but I was ready – I had been waiting for this all summer.

University can be a daunting, yet exciting new experience for so many young adults, however for me it was to be a way of breaking those old habits, freeing me from my restrictions and starting over. Maybe it would even be a time for figuring out who I was behind my bulimia as well?

Unfortunately, I'd convinced myself it would be as easy as just believing in all that. I thought, here I'll be able to work on myself at my own pace and turn my life around! In reality, moving to a new country and starting a demanding course of study, unsurprisingly to me now, played on my anxieties.

At the time it must have been obvious that I did not understand my bulimia at all. I naively thought I had control and was choosing to make myself sick after every meal, because for six years that's what I had convinced myself I wanted and what was best for me. Instead, my bulimia was definitely in charge.

In the early days of my uni experience, I sought comfort in the familiar, now proven-to-work stress-relieving behaviours of bingeing and purging and quick fixes, like alcohol to escape the pressures. This was easy because during freshers' week, and at university in general, anything goes – excessive drinking was almost celebrated! But it quickly got to the point where I did not know who I was without it all. As ridiculous as that may sound now, it was how I'd been dealing with anything and everything that made me uncomfortable, for far too long by that point. Without my bulimia I was weak. Somehow, I had managed to convince myself it was bulimia that made me strong.

I had had every intention of stopping the bingeing and purging and all of the unhealthy behaviours I'd relied on for so long. Instead, I let myself be led by the distractions because it was easier than dealing with myself.

As is more common than perhaps it should be at university, I continued after freshers' week to drink far too much alcohol and dive headfirst into that space where I felt I could truly escape, while sticking rigidly to my extreme internal rules. I binged and purged but I did not feel guilty, alcohol helped numb the pain and it was easy to blame the 'hangover' for anything else I'd be feeling.

At uni, no one knew who I was before, so I could act like the person I wanted to be, the person that fitted in effortlessly; I could keep pretending. Things became so mixed up in my head during this period. I would have thousands of calories from alcohol, but I could not eat a burger or some pasta, fearing the weight gain. I remember going on a date once and ordering a salad alongside a pint of beer – the irrationality!

I made up excuse after excuse to justify my damaging actions, convincing myself it just wasn't the right time to make changes or tackle my issues. *'I need to settle in before I can focus on anything else'* ... *'I need to get going with my studies first'* ... *'It's more important I go to this meal and fit in with a new friendship group than restrict myself'* ... I convinced myself through avoidance that I needed a perfect set of conditions to tackle my issues and it was all too easy to identify the non-perfect conditions that would keep me from making the change, on a daily basis.

It's no surprise to me now that I got into a relationship early on in my uni days, I craved that sense of growing up and recognised on some level that I needed the added external motivation to not be sick. I knew early on, from my relationships with family and friends, that my behaviours were harder to cover up or get away with, if the person I was with cared. Sadly, my first relationship at university was far from ideal and it became very toxic, very quickly.

My boyfriend continuously cheated on me, and I just let it happen. Dealing with it or being distracted by it became another one of my excuses for not making the changes I needed within. Did I blame myself? Did I deserve it? Did

I care? I think, deep down, I put up with it because I was very much aware that I was lying to him and hiding my own secret. Equally, we had no respect for each other, and on top of that, I did not feel worthy or valid of real love because of my secret. I know now that I never actually liked him enough to tell him the truth. He did not deserve to know the real me, but then, I felt no one did. There is no doubt in my mind that so much of what I was feeling internally, was projected into that relationship and I fully accept that that was most likely what he was doing too.

Whatever avoidant behaviour I would adopt or social distraction I would jump into, it was always temporary. And so, somewhat inevitably, when the partying started to get out of hand and the uni work began to stack up, I returned full force to my belief that weight control was the answer to everything. It was the only thing I really cared about. But this time, some part of me started to feel a little scared; maybe I couldn't stop? Maybe this would be my life forever?

During this period, I was still playing international Touch Rugby, but it was a struggle. Almost instinctively, I had joined the gym and started to work out more, doing endless amounts of cardio, and becoming obsessed at seeing the calorie counter go up on the machine I was using. I also started to research ways to speed up my metabolism and for any quick fixes to rid my body of fat. My addictive personality was coming into play again.

Everything I googled, I got answers for... and I was desperate. I needed more quick fixes like fat burner pills or laxatives … anything. It is no wonder the fat loss industry as a whole is one of the most profitable globally, as socially we put everyone under so much pressure about how they look and then provide quick, unhealthy, superficial fixes to a vulnerable audience. The trouble with all that is that people who struggle with their image, including me, don't need to be 'fixed' and certainly not with a lower body weight or body fat percentage.

Aside from the ease of availability, there were no obvious warning signs in purchasing these types of products. I could order multiple quantities of it, to my university address where no one would know or be able to 'catch me'. Deep down, I knew this was unhealthy, but my respect for my body and for myself no longer existed – I was just a vessel for my bulimic thoughts and existence.

I began by taking laxatives, in the popular detox teas that were advertised in *health* shops. This tea is touted as a healthy way to detox and contains ingredients like Mate leaves, which have high levels of flavonoids and antioxidants that are effective for weight loss, and Burdock root, a medicinal herb that works as a laxative. The tea tasted horrid, but I didn't care, it simply did the job. I would drink it eagerly after every meal and then spend an hour or so running back and forth to the toilet with an upset stomach, before revelling in the mild relief of being empty.

I used this tea sporadically for years, always chasing that euphoric feeling of being empty. I also bought green tea pills and synthetic Conjugated Linoleic Acid (CLA) 'fat burners' which have also been widely linked to weight loss. Basically, any fad I happened upon, any quick solution that occurred to me, I'd seize and run with, with no thought of the money I was spending or the damage I was doing to my body; I was spiralling.

Somehow, I got through that first year and then, in my second and third year at university, I had housemates. In my new digs, I continued on as I had before and I'm pretty sure it wasn't too long before my new housemates knew something was going on with me. But, in the same way as my schoolmates, and my roommates at boarding school probably knew, they didn't know how to confront it or me, so instead they took to avoiding it and at times, me. The most reaction I saw was maybe a passive aggressive comment or note from time to time and that suited me. I just saw it all as interference.

I look back at this time and feel a certain sadness. I know I was not a good friend to those around me because I would never allow myself to get close enough to care for anyone or make any real impact. I see the repercussions of that now, with so many of the groups at university staying lifelong friends long into their adult lives. But I had disconnected myself at twelve years old and never let anyone get too close for too many years; it was just too dangerous! I did not trust anyone with my secret, I felt ashamed and scared, but I also did not want anyone's help.

I understand that this must have been a very difficult topic to navigate for my friends. However, I know now that if you recognise that someone is going through some kind of disordered eating in your friendship group, it's essential that it isn't just ignored. My key tip would be to give them the safe space to talk without making them feel like they need to change or that they have a problem. They might not tell you everything straight away, but show them care and concern, without pressure to change. Try to understand what might be fuelling the behaviour as it's unlikely to be as it seems on the surface. Make it about you, make it about what you understand, rather than telling someone what they might be suffering from as there's a good chance they might not know themselves yet. Help them see a different perspective through their disordered lens.

I think so many people were just too fearful to have that conversation with me; they were scared of how negatively I might react (as I would have, not because I was angry but because I was scared). I probably would have convinced them I was fine to the point I would believe it myself (momentarily). This is one of the key underlying motivations I have for wanting to write this book, helping people talk about something that can be scarily common amongst our family and friends yet never spoken about in a raw and honest way. I kept my secret for eight years and even after that I have only shared the bare minimum with people – until now that is.

Chapter Five

NINETEEN

'... eating disorders can become so preoccupying that they virtually take the place of other interpersonal relationships.' Gottlieb, (2023)

What appeared to have been working for me for so long, now felt out of control, but the biggest problem I had was my inability to break the cycle of behaviours trapping me. I was tired, tired of my obsessive and controlling rules and behaviours, and tired of the negativity that consumed me. Tired of going through the motions of life, of not being present or fully connected. I was just so tired.

It was at this point that I recognised I needed help. I was finally able to admit defeat. After seven years, I was now capable of acknowledging that I couldn't fix my issues on my own. There was just no way I could do it alone.

Something deep down inside recognised that this wasn't going to be easy, that reaching out for help might be too tough, so I pivoted and took a seemingly small step towards my recovery journey by buying a £2.99 self-help handbook on Amazon. It was my first and only way of asking for help and by reading it, it got the ball rolling.

Still, the thought of telling someone else was far too tough. I feared judgement and felt shame over my actions having led me to this point. But after buying the book, it was a step I knew I needed to take next, so I hesitantly went to my university counsellor.

I remember the stigma and social apprehension I had on starting therapy. I didn't tell anyone because I was embarrassed; back then, that kind of thing wasn't as talked about as it is today. Now, I will happily advocate for access to therapy for everyone and will continue with it, myself, throughout my adult life because perspective is so important. I find that while I now know a lot of the answers within my subconscious, it's not until I have said them out loud that I listen and act. For me, that's the gift of therapy!

At first, I trod lightly with my counsellor. I lied telling him I had once, in the past, suffered with bulimia but now my issues were *just anxiety*. It helped to test the waters in this way because after eight years, I really didn't know what kind of a reaction I would get when saying my secret out loud. I had never done it before, so I tiptoed on eggshells.

The apprehension in the run up to those appointments was almost excruciating. With each visit, my head spun with a thousand thoughts, not least *Will this counsellor even know how to help me?* At first, I would try to talk honestly and openly, but very quickly, excuses started to crop up, to cover my feelings of shame. Then, little by little, I shared more of my past and current struggles with my counsellor, at a pace that felt safe for me. The only trouble was that these sessions were all too quickly over.

Slowly, my walls were coming down and it was more than terrifying being adrift without the supportive relationship I'd tried to establish with my counsellor. I found myself not knowing what would be left of me without my bulimia: *Who was I?* Bulimia had become such an ingrained part of my everyday life, I would act without thinking; it was second nature, just like brushing my teeth. But I also knew I couldn't continue to live my life from behind those crumbling walls – I was missing out on too much. I had spent too long numb to the world around me.

With time, I began to understand I had been avoiding my emotions using the binge/purge cycle and I knew it would be painful to let myself feel again, every emotion raw. But it wasn't a realistic option to turn away now; I knew life couldn't get any better until I'd gone through it all and life needed to get better.

I felt like I couldn't pretend to put on a brave face anymore, so I dismissed myself from the England touch rugby team to concentrate on getting better, because keeping up with it was all too overwhelming and my lack of fitness was letting my team down. I remember at one of the England camps, before I retreated, we had a nutritionist come in to talk to the group about how to eat correctly for training. For me, this was a reminder that I was in way over my head. I nearly had a breakdown over the amount of carbohydrates we were expected to eat and to top it all off, they wanted us to keep a food diary and monitor our food intake at training. Pure panic ran through my body; I wanted to flee and so when I made the decision, it wasn't as hard as it should have been.

It was around this time that I met Colin (properly). Without knowing, Colin and I had both played in the 2011 Rugby Touch World Cup in Edinburgh. Then, we met properly at mutual friends' wedding in Nottingham. That day, a group of us had arranged to meet at the pub beforehand and he was there. Immediately, I knew he was different. He was a lecturer at Birmingham University and was also completing his PHD, so we would often spend time together in the library as I tried to stay on top of my university assignments. As we spent more time together, we grew closer, and I quickly found he gave me a new kind of hope and external motivation to break free from my bulimia.

Compared to my previous relationships, this time (for the first time), I no longer wanted to be riddled with my bulimia, I did not want to have this secret. I wanted to experience everything for how it really was and not avoid my feelings anymore. But, as I felt myself falling for Colin, I was scared. *How would I be able to maintain my appearance? How could I ever really show my true self to him? I don't want to push him away ...*

At first, when we were together, I would hardly eat, only for me to later binge and purge excessively when he left. When I would eat, I would feel uncomfortable, I'd be trying so hard not to overthink it, but I could feel my body digesting the food and making me feel full. I would torment myself with the idea of dashing to the bathroom to release, but I knew I couldn't as it might ruin everything.

In Colin's absence, I had started to feel guilty when I would stick my fingers down my throat, like I was letting someone down. Suddenly I cared, suddenly I wanted to be normal and not be defined by this illness. I didn't stop though, I just couldn't. Instead, I just suffered even more internal turmoil.

Colin was kind and patient with me, he had been through his own personal journey and provided the safe space I needed at just the right time. I wanted things to work out, more than ever and I knew if I kept such a big secret, we'd never make it. It wasn't fair that I was lying to him.

So, in the same way I did with the counsellor, I slowly broke the truth into pieces, telling him, *"I used to do this,"* then after a while admitting, *"I still sometimes do this,"* until I felt certain he wouldn't turn away. His reactions were always just to listen, to let me talk, and reassure me it didn't change things between us or how he felt about me. I couldn't believe it, in my head, things always went so differently. I always catastrophized that he would leave, that he would say I was disgusting or even worse, force me to stop when I was not ready.

One night Colin and I were talking, and he said the words that I never thought I'd be worthy of hearing; he told me he loved me. I froze, because even though I so desperately wanted to say it back I felt it was not fair to let him say those words when he didn't know the real me, bulimia, and all. So, I told him everything, starting with when I was twelve.

Colin gave me something I had always had from my parents but never realised, unconditional support. He saw me at my worst, the real, vulnerable me, and didn't once turn away. When I told him the biggest, darkest secret that I had held onto for so long and that I was struggling to cope, he helped me and gave me hope and encouraged me to see a different future. A future I wanted for myself too.

Chapter Six

TWENTY

Magnetic resonance imaging (MRI) scans suggest the brains of women with bulimia react differently to images of food after stressful events, when compared with the brains of women without bulimia, American Psychological Association.

I couldn't predict what my future looked like because for eight years now, I had been bulimic and at the age of twenty it was still part of my daily life. I had told Colin how overwhelmed I felt and that I had lost trust in my own judgement and my own ability to recognise and process my emotions; everything that we learn to navigate when we are younger and define throughout our lives. But I wasn't done yet, I needed to tell my parents everything and stop lying to those closest to me, I just didn't know where to start. It felt as if I hardly understood what I was going through, so how could I then vocalise that to the people in this world who cared about me the most?

In the summer, before my final year of university, I told my parents I wasn't going to come back to Malaysia to be with them during the break. I needed the time and space away to get better. I owed it to them, to Colin, and to myself to try. Not being able to be fully honest yet, I gave them an excuse that I needed to get my driving licence and got a job at a sports marketing company for a few weeks to give the impression I was busy.

In the early days, I started to try and understand the 'why' behind what I was doing. *What was I avoiding? Why has this habit controlled me for so long?* There were tears, lots of tears, but over the course of a few weeks, Colin helped me to organise my thoughts and get down on paper what I was going through and what I understood my bulimia to be.

It was finally time to tell my parents the truth, no matter how painful. I knew it was crucial to my recovery journey, as it meant I was no longer holding onto this secret. So, on the 14th of August 2014, I stopped forcibly making myself sick for what I had hoped would be forever, and shortly after, I sent my letter, via email, knowing my choice of not going home was right, as dealing with it in person would be too overwhelming.

The Email:

August 2014

Dear Family,

It is important that I share some very big, personal issues I have been struggling to cope with for a very long time, and I am only just beginning to deal with. I understand this email

will be difficult to read, as it was extremely difficult for me to write.

I know you both, as my parents, love me and are supportive of me. But I also need you to understand there is much more to the problems I am facing than what is on the surface and what you may think or have previously understood.

I have been bulimic for about eight years now. Although you may be aware of this issue from my past, and Mum has tried to catch me out from time to time, the extent to which it has continued and evolved is far worse than what you have thought. Except for very rare occasions I have made myself throw up every single day for the last eight years, often more than once a day.

What is certain is that no one is to blame; my bulimia has progressed and evolved over such a long period of time and for a number of different reasons. I can categorically state it is not simply about food and making myself 'skinny'. Having read extensively about the disorder as part of my healing process and speaking to my counsellor, bulimia is something I have developed as a coping mechanism for all sorts of things and circumstances, such as self-esteem issues and anxious situations. It has become a comforting action and habit, helping me avoid overwhelming tasks and stressful situations—in particular frustration and communication issues. This is something I feel occurs with you, Mum and Dad. As well, it has given me a reason or buffer for failure in tasks and relationships.

What is important is I am finally being completely honest with myself and with you, my family, because I want to fully recover. I am in a better place at the moment than I have been for such a long time. As I have already said, I am seeing a counsellor. But, considering I have been bulimic for eight years, this is a huge step. It is still early stages, but a significant part of my recovery is making you, as my family, aware. Colin and you three are the only ones that know and are the only ones that will know. I am not doing this for attention. It is about confronting triggers/causes and issues that fuel the disorder.

First as I said above, the fact that I am even able to write this email is a huge factor and a massive step in my recovery. But as my bulimia developed and continued for eight years it is not simply going to stop overnight. This summer I've had time and I've been on my own to properly deal with it once and for all. This means diving deep and understanding what has caused it, going back to when it all started and assessing the changes from being at Alice Smith to now being at uni. This will fully help me to understand why it has continued for so long. As I alluded to above, it has only really been in the last month that I have understood about 80% of the actual disorder, and the lengths required to fix what is causing my bulimia and understanding what has caused it for so long. Before that I was naive to the point where although at times I wanted to stop, I simply thought it was an overnight process and was something I could turn off. Doing something as simple as buying a recovery guide and help book only happened at the beginning of this summer.

Through this email I am going to help you to understand what have been the causes and underlying motivations behind the disorder. This does not mean I am putting the blame for this on anyone. I am simply making you all aware that a massive part of the development of my bulimia has been family-related issues. So, however you feel at the end of this email, please don't feel bad. I am in a better place and am finally moving past it all. Half of the causes have been unintentional or progressed over time because of my own mindset in seeing and dealing with particular situations. Although these may involve you, it is not anyone's fault. A lot of this is the past. If I can move on, 'forgive and forget', you need to as well. I need you to not get angry with me, as you have done in the past.

From the book: "Bulimia often begins as an innocent attempt to protect thinness and thus please others. The person with bulimia is not following her own heart; she is reacting to what's going on around her. It appears to be protecting her by preserving a false front and a sense of safety, whilst keeping people at a distance. Bulimics interact with people knowing they can withdraw to their repetitive familiar behaviours at any time. Bulimics maintain a happy, competent façade on the outside, while feeling anxious or depressed on the inside. Mood swings are common (HA … I think I would still have these). Bulimics are often considered confident, outgoing and independent people, presenting an acceptable front when they are insecure underneath.

Remember an eating disorder is not just about food, food is used as a method of control".

I am happy to answer any questions you may have. Like I say, I have a recovery book which I've read and found extremely helpful in understanding bulimia myself as I—until recently—was unaware of the extent to which this has taken control over my own life. If anyone wants to read the book to know more you are welcome to, as sharing this secret has also relieved a considerable amount of pent-up emotions which I have bottled up for years. Now you are all aware I feel if I need to communicate certain things, I hope that you can be much more understanding, and I much calmer in telling you.

"Eating disorders are feeling disorders. The rigid rules and rituals of bulimic behaviour are a definite way to distance oneself from feelings that seem unmanageable, overwhelming or just plain terrifying. Eventually bulimics find no other way to handle their feelings except to binge and purge – 'powerless'. These unvoiced feelings, find an expression in other ways".

In the very beginning and early stages of this disorder I used purging to reach a low weight. However, bulimia provided a false sense of self-esteem, competence, and control. Later on, the disorder provided a mental numbness and physical high making it very addictive. Impulsive behaviours are consequences/side effects of bulimia. I used to get drunk A LOT when I was fifteen/sixteen/seventeen. I also smoked. I also shoplifted. I also 'fought the system' at boarding school – in hindsight and with my understanding of bulimia these were all cries for attention.

"Parents of bulimics especially need to beware of their limitations in helping their children. Often the relationship is too close for objective evaluation. Parents usually play a part in the development of their child's behaviour and in many instances have to face issues and make adjustments of their own. This is not to say they are the cause of the eating disorder but that they may have contributed to it in some way and need to acknowledge that. Parents need to re-evaluate feelings/ways of communicating, ways of handling feelings/parenting roles and decision making within the family".

For years and years, I had built up in my head that throwing up was something I felt forced to do as a way of controlling my body/image. However, since boarding school and university where my daily routine and food intake is completely of my own choosing, I have now come to realise it is so much more. After numerous failed attempts to stop I realised it is not something I could simply turn off. Having read extensively about it and been to see the counsellor, it has taken me eight years to say, "I have bulimia," out loud and although I have always known I have had this problem I have never felt the need to change or fully get better.

Imagine carrying a massive secret that affects your daily routine so extensively every day for eight years – especially a secret as big as this and one which you have to hide from all your friends and family. As a result of this, the majority of my friendships and relationships (prior to Colin) have been somewhat fake and a visage on the surface. I know you have not met Colin. To you it may be another relationship. But Colin is the first person that I have felt I could be completely honest with and open up with about this, as well the first person I have wanted to be fully honest with. Although it has taken its toll on me, I am grateful that I am finally accepting it all by being honest and putting in the work to fully recover. Colin has supported me and motivated me to live a healthier/ happier and more fulfilling life. So, whatever you think, he is an extremely important person in my life. You, as my family, should be grateful that he has helped me to be completely honest with myself and with you.

I do not wish for this message to come across as ungrateful. I have had an incredible life and childhood. Please do not be sad or feel sorry for me. Unfortunately, yes, this disorder has consumed a massive part of my childhood. But it does not mean I am not grateful and have not experienced life for the last eight years. To be where I am now, I am extremely fortunate. I love you very much.

I am sorry I did not come to both of you as I know you have always been there to help me and love me. This circumstance was different. The eating disorder has been used as my way of dealing with a lot of emotions and anxieties. One main source of emotion and anxiety is with you both and Sam, and how I feel I have to act in terms of our family dynamics. I developed this coping strategy of bulimia to avoid dealing with other issues as well, which started when I was extremely young. Although my weight did regulate the issue of my bulimia has only gotten worse. There is no straight answer to why people become bulimic. However, from what I understand bulimia is considered to be a psychological and emotional disorder. People become addicted to the behaviour to avoid painful feelings/pressures/low self-esteem (you always said I had an addictive personality …).

I am sharing all of this with you so that I don't have to carry the secret anymore, and for your support. You cannot imagine the weight that is being lifted from simply writing this all out. Although there is not much you can physically do to help my recovery, do not underestimate how much simply being aware will help me, as it is allowing me to be honest. The holiday in Italy will be a risky situation for me as the relapse rate for bulimia is extremely high. It will be a lot easier if you are all in understanding with me and on the same page. If I feel tense or a problem arises, I am hoping I can openly talk to you about it, rather than go back to my secretive ways that I know far too well.

We can all agree I have struggled to 'communicate' with you both over a number of things throughout my life because I often get overly emotional and feel frustrated. Please don't patronise me, or think you know best in this situation. It is something I am dealing with on my own and because of the nature of this, this is how it has to be. This is something I know much more about than you do. I know, Mum, you may feel helpless in Malaysia but in reality, as I am at uni and I live on my own I need to get better on my own as I need to take responsibility and care of myself. At the end of the day, I am the only one that can help myself and I now finally realise that. My anxiety/driving failures/IB grades etc have all been directly related to this. Although I went to the counsellor to discuss my anxiety issues, we have spent the entire time slowly dissecting and understanding my disorder.

I am at the point with myself now that it doesn't matter what has happened in the past or how things may have affected me. Of course, nothing and none of this was intended but I am explaining the harsh reality of how certain circumstances and situations in the past have affected me more than you could have imagined. Because this started when I was so young, it is only now I can fully work through it all. At twelve/thirteen, I did not think logically or rationally as I was a young child. It is however not too late to finally correct it all.

What was originally used as a method of control has developed into something that I found I was out of control of. My reasons for not sharing this with you or for keeping this secret for so long is that mostly I've been afraid. When I was twelve/thirteen, and this all started and it was obvious as I dropped to 44 kg, I agree I looked ill. I remember the day you both confronted me about this. We were at the cheap Chinese restaurant in Sri Hartamas and you both got angry at me and shouted, "What's wrong with you, you look ill etc., etc.." This caused me to develop my fear of speaking to you. I was so young and clearly suffering from a serious illness, and in my own messed up way was screaming for help. You guys responded by getting angry at me. Mum, I know you tried to help me and offered for us to get rid of this together or I would have to seek professional help in Malaysia. However, we never really spoke about my problems. It was simply about my weight. Your offering to seek professional advice was perceived by me as a threat. I was not ready, and this terrified me. Therefore, I got my weight up so that to you both I appeared to be recovered. However, the secrecy and the throwing up continued. I know you were worried and scared for my health, but I didn't know any better and was just as afraid. You should not have got angry at me because that just scared me into keeping it a secret and hiding it from you. I was twelve. But this is in the past. That was only the beginning. This has since then continued to develop over the years, as I got very good at hiding this secret and used to go to great lengths to do so.

I used to 'go for a run' and make myself throw up so Mum wouldn't smell sick in my bathroom as you used to continuously try and catch me out. Again, confronting me in an angry way made me more scared and more determined to keep it from you both. This then developed to me feeling the most insecure and on edge in front of my own family. Being in a bikini around you is the worst thing for me. I feel so uncomfortable. I feel like I am constantly being judged. My environment and a number of things have changed over time (home/boarding school/uni) but our relationship and built-up frustrations that I have about communicating and keeping this a secret have remained constant.

Sam, I love you to bits. When I was younger you were my

role model (believe it or not!); as my older brother I wanted to be just like you. Sam, you were skinny when you were younger and could eat whatever you wanted. I was not fat, but I still had "puppy fat" or whatever you want to call it and could not understand why we would eat the same amount, but you were always smaller than me. I try so hard when I am around you because I feel like my body/look is constantly being judged. If you say I look nice it's a massive thing for me. This is in combination with you going through all the life steps first and succeeding. This put so much pressure on me, in regard to getting good IB grades, getting into a good uni (two things I struggled massively with). The pressures from this have helped fuel my disorder; for me it numbs the stress of it all. It also gave me an excuse for failing. Luckily, I am fortunate to be at a good university.

You can think I'm being harsh or being unreasonable or unrealistic about these things, but they have all affected me to the point of being ill for eight years. I think that justifies me attempting to explain to you where some of this has stemmed from and for you to listen. As a family we all have strong personalities that clash. You often make me feel really difficult. A small example (from many)—in Cheltenham in September, the simple event of Sam wanting to go to an Indian restaurant. This is coupled with your general tendency Sam, to plan everything around meals (especially when Mum and Dad are paying), and then interpret me not getting excited as not wanting to spend time with the family. I do want to spend time with my family. It is just that it is incredibly difficult for me to eat meals outside of certain places. I then have to make excuses to hide this, and then the rest of the family reacts in a very negative way.

Mum, when I was in Malaysia, I wouldn't go out with you and eat all the nice Asian lunches, like Sam would. You then kept going on about this. You may have been joking, but as I perceive it, it was hurtful. I need you to be more empathetic and understanding of my condition, and just think about how things may affect people. Words hurt, as I am sure I have accidently upset you guys in the past. But you making me feel difficult meant that in order not to come across as difficult, I would then be sick. It was easier to just go and then deal with it how I knew best. I have always been trying to keep you guys happy. I now need to be selfish for my own health. I need you to stop comparing me to Sam. Everybody is different. It is these small things that mean my frustrations have progressed over the years to the extent where I now cannot have a serious conversation with you all without crying and getting extremely emotional.

I do not want to repeat myself, but a lack of independence is a cause. Again, this is no one's fault, but these circumstantial influences have contributed to my illness. Whilst it may now be too late, I did not understand when I was younger why Sam was allowed to do more things than I was. Yes, now it is obvious; he is a boy and older. But back then it just made me frustrated. Boarding school, which was then to me 'prison' fuelled those frustrations even more and made my eating/throwing up worse. Dad, I know I will always be 'your little girl' but you cannot expect everything to go your way. I have grown up believing that you do not listen to me, do not understand me, or take me seriously. Finally—and this is the last time I am going to say it, and it is a minor point—please stop talking about meeting Colin. When I want you to and the timing is right you will. It is my (and his!) choice.

Sam, I love you and you are living your life to the full but don't tell me what I should be doing at university because I'm not going out or going on holidays every weekend. It is my university life. Let me live it how I want to. For me what is more important than anything right now is getting better so that I can complete the final year healthy and happy and to the best of my ability. Drinking negatively impacts it. It is why I don't feel confident going out loads anymore.

Before you reply, please take your time, and please do not be hurt. The email is simply for you to be aware. I am not looking for help or for sympathy; I just want you to try and understand. No one could have known it would get to be this bad. I didn't even really know what was going on, as for a long time I thought it was only about being skinny and that was all I cared about but when I tried to stop numerous times about five years ago, I found I couldn't.

I know I am recovering. It has been an extremely difficult few months as with anything it gets worse before it gets better but writing this now it's getting better. The majority of this email talks about things that are in the past. So, things are looking up already. If you do not know how to respond to this

email, then sit and think about it a little longer. Alternatively, we can talk when I next see you. See you in September.

Xxxxxxxxxxxx

My parents were in shock. They had known of my struggles, but not of the depths of them and the words I'd struggled to write, hit them as it would any parent, hard. They thought I had been rid of this for years and did not have any idea that it had continued, secretly, for so many years.

I didn't feel like I could speak to my parents, after sending the email, not in person, nor on the phone: I was afraid of how to continue life without my coping mechanism. Every day was a battle to come to terms with things I'd buried deep down and to resist the quick fix behaviours I'd relied on, and I just didn't have it in me to be that vulnerable yet. We did email back and forth, keeping the communication going and that made it easier in the short term, but I felt like I had let them down, and at the same time like they would never understand. How could they?

Then, in September, we had a family holiday to Italy that had been booked for months. It was my chance to face my parents. Ordinarily, I would have so enjoyed this uninterrupted time with them and the wonders that Italy is blessed with. And in an effort to make it so, I'd planned ahead and prepared my family for the space I'd need, going forward but at this stage I was not aware of what I needed and how I would cope. The reality of my situation (being in the early days of my recovery), meant we were at odds for most of the holiday. My parents were desperate to enjoy every moment and I was desperate to just hold on. I think back and feel mixed emotions of that holiday, I know I was so difficult and hard to have around, and it is not that I did not appreciate being on holiday in such a beautiful country, I was just in a very different head space and the basics of everyday were hard but it was good for me. I had to force myself into environments like these as it was the only way.

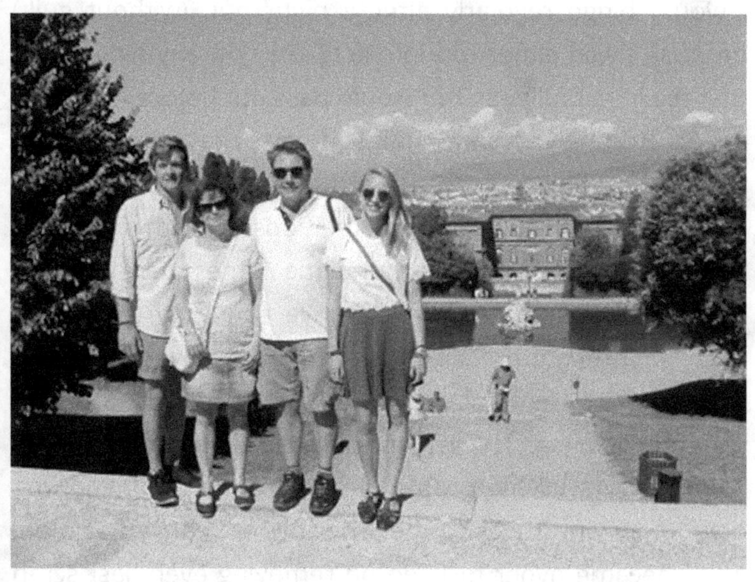

Family photo in Florence, September 2014

When I returned to Loughborough as university started back from the summer break, my days looked the same. I found the only solace I could get was keeping to a strict routine: One day at a time.

Despite my progress, I still monitored my weight, constantly checking my reflection in the mirror and staring at my stomach, as if one meal would dramatically change my appearance. Daily, I kept a paper diary and recorded all my meals, which consisted of no more than 500 calories. There were no carbs allowed, still, and I used chewing gum to keep me going between meals. My lack of understanding was shown by the fact I was still drinking, and not just vodka sodas but sweet, calorific fruit ciders. During this period, I would binge regularly after a night out, (without guilt) because I was either too intoxicated to do anything about that feeling of fullness, or I would pass out before I could.

Frustratingly, despite the good news that I had stopped being sick, I had to come to terms with the fact that I still had an extremely unhealthy relationship with food and some of my behaviours around mealtimes were still too negative. I was so far from intuitive eating by that point, because it meant breaking every rule I had lived by since I could properly remember; the going was tough!

One evening, I recall making dinner with Colin. He would always let me cook and prepare the food, knowing how important it was to me. That night, I cooked salmon, and I became hyper focused on removing every last scrap of the fatty skin from the fillet. I was so driven, to the extent that I became frustrated and hysterical, screaming over the futility of it all – that wasn't unusual and thankfully, neither was Colin's patience.

I fought with myself every day not to give in to the relentless urge to release the pressures of life, by purging. I was constantly at breaking point as I tried to come to terms with changing my behaviours around food and mealtimes. I struggled to process anything rationally. For example, I would not eat pasta because of the carb content, but I ate sweets more than anything because I was always hungry and several times a week, I still drank to get drunk, because I needed the escape. I would frequently have dreams that I had relapsed, waking up with a pit in my stomach that all this pain had been for nothing.

There were so many rules in my head around that time, that I did not know what was factual and what was a product of my illness. But I got through university and concentrated on trying my best not to repeat the mistakes I made during my final exams at school. Colin, undertaking his PHD, often studied with me and became my safe haven. I could stay with him, concentrating on my coursework and knowing I had someone watching over me in terms of my behaviour patterns with food. I owe so much to him because I know I was not easy to be around and so much of my pent-up and frustrated behaviour would have not made sense and been transferred onto him.

What he did so well is that he never questioned me, never judged me for my behaviours with food, or by the amounts I would eat. He listened to and supported me, allowing me to recover in my own time, gradually, in a safe space over the next couple of years. It was not linear, but his support was constant. Colin would pick me up when I did not have the strength.

After finishing university, I moved to Birmingham on a graduate scheme in Commercial Property where Colin lived and worked. We moved in together and while I never told him this, I vowed never to binge and purge in our home. It was another example of the rules I created, but this time I knew it was a good one. It would be a clean break. I could not break his trust and I did not want to let him down. I also did not want the place we lived to be associated with my illness. So, I began working full time, while completing my Real Estate Masters, part time, being busy made it a little easier.

I found living together a little tough, at first, it was so different from when I was at university, where I had housemates but still full independence. However, I knew it was absolutely an important part of my recovery. Committing to never performing those behaviours in that environment was an exercise in self-discipline and inner strength and I grew stronger every day. I found being accountable to someone, other than myself, difficult, but we each understood and were there for each other.

Around this time, my parents bought a flat in Cheltenham and I had planned to go home and spend time with them there for Easter. Plus, I figured, it would give

Colin a break. After reading my email and some thorough searching, my mum had found a world-renowned eating disorder therapist, Dr Kirsten, and had managed to make an appointment for me, for when I was with them. This was another pivotal moment for me and the catalyst I needed to get beneath the surface of what was driving my bulimia and continue my journey of recovery. My parents, after seeing how much I was still suffering every day, and trying to keep my job, degree and relationship together, offered their support in the best way they could.

Immediately, I felt at ease talking with my new therapist because I'd already reached a point where I was receptive to the advice of others. If I hadn't, I don't know if she could have broken down my barriers, or even if I'd have ever made it there to meet her. But I wanted out now, I wanted to understand, and I finally felt I could open and not be too crushed by disappointment and judgement.

I was forced to look at myself, and I mean really look. The only way I was going to really understand and get better was to go back to the beginning.

One of the first things I realised was that, like a lot of people, I had a real lack of education around food, instead I had spent years living by my own (well portrayed to me by the media), socially constructed beliefs and had never associated the food in front of me, with what my body needed physically. That was something I could easily fix.

Despite my sporting background, I had a fundamental fear of carbs, I didn't understand energy input vs output and what a body required. My version of the food groups was simply categorised as good or bad. Then, through talking, I began to see the relevance of things, where I hadn't before; I was able to think about things from a different perspective. A whole new world began to open up before me and finally, things started to make sense – I was not avoiding life anymore. I learnt about maintenance calories and what your body requires on a daily basis just to live, to breathe, to have healthy and normal brain function.

Thanks to my therapist, I felt seen in a way that I hadn't before, despite my friends and family having tried. The timing, along with her specialist knowledge, left me feeling safe and her patience put me at ease. Going into her office, it had been nearly eight months of not making myself sick, and one of the biggest things she did for me was to praise my efforts to stop the binge/purge cycle. I hadn't allowed myself the space to stop and see what I had done so far, nor taken the time to congratulate myself on my progress, because of all the noise still in my head. She said, *'Well Done!'* and it meant everything.

My therapist helped me to see I'd been 'firefighting' for most of my life. Any time an issue arose, I would deal with it in my way, mostly avoiding those issues. Obviously, this takes an emotional toll and that's where the familiarity and reliability of my food-related behaviours came in. I internalised everything, I was the problem. When I began to feel too different, I blamed my weight. When I felt pressured to be like the others, in a social context or stressed by my exams, worried about anything, I blamed my appearance. It was a pattern of avoidance.

She also helped to examine my competitive nature and analyse the unhelpful comparisons I'd been forever making with others, especially with my brother. I had always idolised my brother, who at three years my senior, seemed to have it all going on, and that meant I wanted to be like him. I always watched him being adventurous, outgoing, full of confidence, and seemingly successful in every endeavour. Then I'd think about me being overly self-critical and overthinking everything. I remember being afraid to go up against him in any proper competitions, because he'd always win; the way I did compete, was in my head. I'd been constantly comparing myself to things that were not comparable.

I learned that I reached out for control in a world where I felt I didn't have any. I had been susceptible to the media, to magazines and pop culture's depictions of beauty. I bowed under cultural and traditional expectations, to those habits prevalent in my own home, and to peer pressure.

I acknowledged that my chosen method had always been to withdraw and internalise, because the only voice I trusted was my own, and this had only got worse as I had got older. That created an almost impenetrable barrier, which only now was coming down. But it took a while for everything to fall into place. I was learning and, on my way, to recognising that my internal voice is capable of being compassionate to me, if I really needed it to be.

Therapy set me on track for completing my master's degree and graduate scheme in Birmingham then I moved to London to continue with my company in a new role. I spent the next five years coping with work, with my relationship, and with my international touch rugby. I had completed my master's degree and chartered surveying qualification, moved to London to pursue my commercial property career and lived in Clapham with my best friend from university. Everything was good, I was good. I had faced a lot of my fears and was rebuilding myself. My relationship with my parents was also something that I began to cherish now that the darker days were behind me. Ever since boarding school I had got into the habit of calling them every other day or so and keeping communication going regularly to make up for the distance between us. Mum became my best friend again because I was no longer shutting her out.

Mine and Colin's relationship stayed strong through this period and spanned over six years. I will forever be grateful for our time together and for the support and love we gave each other. He saw me at my absolute worst, trying to regulate and process my emotions and struggling daily with my rigid rules, as I started to feel the emotions I'd suppressed for so long. He remained patient and stayed by my side, giving me the courage to finally say my secret out loud. I believe our stories were not written for us to be together forever, but today, Colin and I remain friends and I'll never forget all that he did for me and for helping me to write that email, because I could not have done it on my own.

Chapter Seven

TWENTY-FIVE

'Relapse rates for clients successfully treated for bulimia nervosa range from 31% to 44% during the first two years of recovery.' Very Well mind.com (2023)

In 2019, I'd been reselected to play and, this time captain the England mixed open team at the Touch Rugby World Cup which was being hosted in Malaysia. This was an absolute honour for me and to be able to go back home to play was exciting too!

Work took a bit of a back seat around this time, as the midweek training and weekend camps for the world cup became a big commitment. I didn't mind though; it was nice to have something to work towards and focus all my energies into, plus I did always like being busy.

Unfortunately, I became complacent. I believed, after five years of not making myself sick, that I had recovered. I no longer used it as my coping mechanism which to me meant that I did not have bulimia anymore. *Surely, I was fixed?*

What I hadn't noticed, was that small habits had started to reform. I began by tracking my calories, weighing myself daily, and constantly checking my stomach in the mirror. I quickly began letting a 'fat day' dictate my mood and above all else, I fell back into being constantly critical of myself.

The World Cup gave me plenty of excuses for overtraining. My addictive (and disciplined), personality thrived, and I quickly developed orthorexia, an obsession with excessive exercising. I stopped drinking all alcohol and dramatically reduced my socialising too. Instead, I used 'MyFitnessPal' for everything I ate, even down to a thirteen-calorie corn cake. Often, I would overeat because I was so hungry, then I would 'cheat', by logging the extra food I'd eaten in the section for the day after, which soon developed into a vicious cycle. At work I ate no 'treats' when it was someone's birthday, or when the treat trolley came around on a Friday; *I can't, I am training for the World Cup,* I would say.

It was all too easy to slip back towards my dangerous behaviours. Because of the World Cup, I didn't need convincing to exercise and restrict myself; it was all absolutely necessary, and the obsessiveness was simply because I cared about representing my country. I was a dedicated athlete!

I took satisfaction from the fact that no one would question what I was doing. Even over the Christmas holidays (four months after the tournament), while on holiday in Thailand, I was waking up early and completing my fitness sessions. I had convinced myself, so I truly believed I was at my 'healthiest'.

In reality, I was spiralling into a different version of my eating disorder, and I had found a new form of escapism.

Things got worse. People would tell me how good and fit and healthy I looked, and how dedicated I was, essentially validating what I was doing to myself. Of course, they weren't to know, but their compliments just made me even more obsessive about training. I had abs, because I was undereating, and I definitely started to enjoy the compliments too much. Not only was I looking 'good', I was more confident in myself, loving this new version of me and feeling proud that I had found a way to be lean, without making myself sick. It did not matter that it was not sustainable.

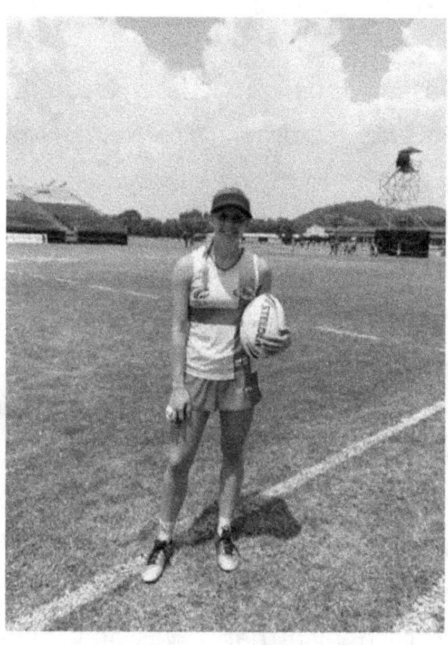

Touch Rugby World cup in Malaysia, April 2019

When the World Cup came around it was such a proud time for me and a core memory I will never forget. For the five days of the tournament, I thought about nothing else. I was so present with the team, fully immersed and dedicated to each game we played; I felt alive, just taking it all in.

But when it finished, while tournament blues are a normal thing, I experienced an extreme case. I started to feel a bit lost; I just didn't know who I was supposed to be anymore. I didn't know what to do with the time I'd dedicated to my training, and worse, I no longer had the external motivation of the tournament to keep me on track with my goals. Slowly, I began to realise that I had sacrificed and changed so much in my life towards a tournament that was now over.

Now, I was anxious about how I could continue my ongoing habits without drawing criticism. How could I stay lean? I liked how I felt in my new body.

I think it was at this moment I finally accepted that a huge part of my story with bulimia was centred around my addictive personality. I was constantly swapping my focus towards external events or people in my life, in an attempt to avoid my deep-down insecurities and feelings towards myself. While bulimia was my key coping mechanism, it didn't fix anything, so that when I stopped physically being sick, all of the underlying causes were still there; my output was just different.

I began to recognise that it was only a matter of time before all the distractions would stop working. I had focused so much on the goal of not being sick in 2014, that I saw that success as the key indicator that I was better. I didn't ever take the time to realise my thought patterns and behaviours around food had never really changed.

Unsurprisingly, a few months after the World Cup, it all became too much. I was doing fine at work, but I didn't see my job as a career, because I was focused on trying to move back to Asia – another form of escapism no doubt. Similarly, my relationship had been coasting along, with me in London and Colin now in Leicester; he had his own things to focus on, and at this time he needed to be there for himself. I felt isolated and overwhelmed and it was all depressingly familiar.

Despite this, I still wanted to hold on to being lean for as long as possible. Fundamentally, I did not want to put on weight, I wanted to stay that shape forever. Then, I got too drunk on a night out, and all too easily made myself sick, promising myself it would be just the once, because I had overeaten.

And then I made myself sick at work. This time it was because I couldn't refrain from the treats that were being handed out and for months, I had restricted myself from eating anything 'sweet' because of the World Cup. Now, it was an excuse I could not use anymore and in the absence of another, I reverted back to what I knew would work for me: I felt incredibly weak.

Soon, it became a couple of times a month that I'd make myself sick, but before long it increased to twice a week. The terrifying thing was just how good it felt in the immediate aftermath. I remembered straight away that euphoric feeling of relief, the feeling of accomplishment, and there really was no other feeling like it!

I realised then that it never goes away. Once you've been there, felt that, lived this, you just have to find a way to manage it.

On the other hand, I can still remember the anxious feelings I felt afterwards, in the quiet. The opposing voices competed in my head for prominence and up against my bulimia was such a vast amount of crushing disappointment when I realised, I was still suffering with this mental illness, and it really would be a part of me forever. I knew I'd ended up in a dangerous place again and I would have to work hard to get out. Thankfully, I knew I wasn't starting from the complete beginning, thanks to my earlier efforts, but there was still so much I did not understand about my bulimia.

Ultimately, I felt that I had failed myself and, frankly, I was embarrassed to be in my mid-twenties and still controlled by this illness. It had been shamefully easy to fall back into old habits, as I'd naively thought my sessions with the counsellor in Cheltenham were all I needed to take me forward in life. Here, I felt that, even though she'd given me some much-needed insight and the tools to work with, on my own, for someone who was so disciplined, I had gotten so lazy with myself and with my own recovery.

I realised I needed help (again), but I was far too distressed to tell anyone close to me, so I booked in to see another counsellor through my private health insurance at work. I had six sessions granted to me and the first one was especially hard, going back to the beginning, repeating the same story I had told so many times and thought I would not have to repeat again. But, before I knew it, the last session came around and I had not even touched the surface. I found I had just repeated all the understanding I had gleaned from previous years. *Was I fixed?* Of course not.

Chapter Eight

TWENTY-SIX

Patients presenting with conditions such as anorexia and bulimia were found to have been thriving in the isolation of lockdown during the COVID-19 pandemic.
Ayton (2022)

I saw the numbers of sick and dying people rising alarmingly, all over the world, on the news reports. The COVID-19 pandemic would go on to change the world, but I had my own struggles to deal with.

In March 2020 I had said goodbye to the only place I had ever worked, as I had been there since I was a graduate. I had managed to navigate a move back to Singapore, by joining a Singaporean company with commercial property in London. And then, in the middle of all that the world went into lockdown.

Colin and I had reached an unhealthy stage in our relationship. A stage that grew out of empathy and understanding, but sadly turned into more of a codependency, than a romantic love. I felt that we both relied on each other being a distraction, to avoid facing our own realities. On top of that, my move back to Asia was not something I was willing to compromise on.

At first, we tried to find Colin opportunities out there too, but it was not meant to be. During that time, Colin needed me more and more, and I was finding it hard to keep up; I had so much work still to do for myself. We knew that we loved each other still, but we soon realised we needed to go our separate ways and support each other by giving one another the space and strength to face our own battles, in the scariest way imaginable, without each other.

The pandemic was hard to process, especially on my own. It was an uncertain time, where things were constantly changing, and no one knew how it would unfold. The place I was in on my personal journey, meant I was not strong enough to cope with the extra trauma; I don't think many were, to be honest. Uncertainty can be terrifying especially for someone like me who loves a plan as much as keeping busy in the gym.

At the time, of the first lockdown I was living in Clapham with my housemate who had been seconded to work for a company that set up COVID testing sites. I had already started my new job and was gearing up for my move at the end of summer, as soon as my work visa had come through for Singapore. Despite my turmoil, I was becoming excited for this next chapter and a fresh start.

For me, the first lockdown was all about surviving. I

quickly developed routines that included bedroom HIIT workouts, park runs and basically keeping as active (and therefore as calm), as possible. I got seriously into running, and honestly tried to form more healthy habits, which helped to keep my mind occupied. But I was in unfamiliar territory, so I used the calorie burn function on my Apple watch, tracking every session I could, simply to try and keep accountable.

Still, the boredom threatened to trigger those overwhelming feelings and I didn't know what else to do to keep them at bay when my housemate left to set up testing sites, and I found myself alone. There was so much volatility with the pandemic, and it was looking ever more likely to threaten my move to Singapore. My feelings of desperation grew and before long, I found myself reverting back to my inner child, making myself sick for the relief, for the break, for the boredom.

When we came out of that first lockdown, in Summer 2020, I was still adjusting to not having Colin in my life every day, which wasn't easy. I hadn't tried to live this way on my own before, so the lack of accountability and easily available support frightened me. I also knew that, if my move could go ahead, I had one last summer in London, which, after being in lockdown for months, had to be a good one!

That summer, I said yes to everything; alcohol, drugs, partying ... I did not have any touch rugby to play and keep my fitness on track, and I also did not have a boyfriend to spend time with and keep me accountable. In the moment,

I had the time of my life and I remember everyone around me kept saying how fun I was and how happy I seemed. I even convinced myself that I was, that I was having so much fun; it was very much a *YOLO* mentality.

The reality was that I was miserable; my mental health was being severely neglected. I just stopped acknowledging the work I needed to do and settled into avoidance again: I wanted to escape from my own reality, and it was far easier to do than living it.

When the second lockdown hit, I was in a bad place. My move to Singapore had to be delayed due to COVID and I was devastated. I had convinced myself that when I got on the plane, I would be able to forget everything and start over. I was deluded about how much I was really suffering. To make matters worse, I'd given up my tenancy in Clapham and was forced to move into a new temporary apartment in Canary Wharf for a couple of months, while a new visa came through. I was extremely grateful for this beautiful, one bedroom apartment, the problem was that it meant I was isolated and alone (again), and I knew that my self-destructive behaviours would continue: I had no fight left in me.

Looking back now, it was clear that, although it had been the best decision for both of us in the long term, I had not adequately dealt with my breakup with Colin. This played on my mind, and I withdrew from myself and allowed my addictive tendencies to run riot. In trying to work from home and keep the new job going in a completely new working environment, I turned to obsessively picking at my skin, leaving scars all over my face and having to take numerous rounds of antibiotics to deal with infections. It wasn't long before I stopped leaving the house altogether, which wasn't too bad. Because of the lockdown everyone was struggling, everyone was away from family. I felt like I was not in any way special and so I refused to ask for help.

I was headed down a very dark path by October of that year. The pain I was feeling was the worst it had been. Towards the end, I was being sick several times a week again and my distraction behaviours and need to seek immediate fixes, were all too overwhelming. I was going to the Tesco opposite my building and stocking up on binge food, only to put my head down the toilet an hour later. It became a new way of wasting hours in my day.

In November time, I found I couldn't hide it anymore. I broke down on the phone to my mum and told her the state I was in, even though I think she could already see it for herself. This was essential for me to do; if I had learnt anything from last time, it was not to wait years to ask for help! When I spoke on that call, I was beyond breaking point and desperate.

In December, after twelve months of not seeing her (and despite covid restrictions and difficulties), my mum flew to the UK, and I will forever be grateful that she did. She helped me to save me.

Sometimes it takes admitting defeat, admitting you are not strong enough, and that you can't do it alone to get to where you need to be. I dare not think of what might have happened, had my mum not come over; luckily that's not how my story goes.

On the 30th of November, two days before she arrived, with the hope that I would no longer have to do another lockdown alone, I made myself sick for the last time ever.

Chapter Nine

TWENTY-SEVEN

'There are five Stages of Change that occur in the recovery process: Pre-Contemplation, Contemplation, Preparation, Action, and Maintenance.' National Eating Disorders Organisation, "2023)

As humans we can make things so complex that it makes it harder to understand, or means we avoid understanding all together ...

On the 1st of December 2021, I began my recovery journey for the 100th time on paper, but in reality, for the first time, properly.

This time I had the unwavering support of my mum, who was also supporting her poorly father at that time and was on the other side of the world from my dad and her home, in a global pandemic: Superwoman!

But what I thought had been my lowest point in 2014, had simply been a practice run. Everything about it felt different this time. It felt worse, I think, because I had been given a horrible taste of the reality that bulimia is not something you just overcome or be rid of, it's something to be understood and worked on every day.

So, when the whole world existed in panic and the UK went into its third lockdown, I seized my second chance. Without distraction and with my mum by my side, I very slowly peeled away the layers and built myself back up, little by little. Every day, I was learning a whole new set of habits to take forward for the rest of my life. And I told myself, each day, all I needed to do was be better than the day before.

Mum stayed in the apartment next door to mine for six weeks and we enjoyed the most precious period of bonding time we've ever had. It was beautiful, just the two of us, enjoying each other's company and re-learning about each other. I even started to enjoy mealtimes for the first time, as we got into cooking together using HelloFresh packs. It was the simple things like a glass of wine and a game of scrabble (which I always lost), that I was so grateful to be in the moment for. That time was for really taking things back to basics, but above all I felt safe, and I had the support I needed.

Finding enjoyment in the cooking and sharing of meals together was a revelation for me and not something I had ever felt before. Soon, I felt a strong desire to be able to enjoy food in my future, because I could see that all along it was never about the food. It was what the food was used as that was always the problem; control and release. I accepted that now.

I was still looking forward to my move to Singapore,

although there was still no set date yet. Then, one evening after dinner with Mum, I went back to my apartment and downloaded Hinge, the dating app. I was curious, if anything, as I had never been on a dating app before; when Tinder first came out, I was already in a relationship. It wasn't that I felt ready for a new relationship, and I definitely wasn't looking as there was no point, when I was moving to the other side of the world, and it was lockdown ... Besides, I was still needing to focus on myself and would need to be careful not to jeopardise that. I went on the app a few times, often deleting, or never replying to conversations because I just was not that interested.

One night, towards the end of January, after co-incidentally saying to my mum over dinner that I thought I might be over my previous relationship and feel in a good place, I returned to my apartment, and I matched with Joseph on Hinge. I always think it's funny how these things work out and how beautiful a thing like timing can be. Straight away, I knew it was different with him.

Joseph was honest from the start and told me about his personal story; he had his own struggle with addiction and was also on a journey of recovery. Admittedly, I did not know what to think at first, naively I thought when he said he did not drink it was because he was into CrossFit (like I had stopped drinking for six months when training for the World Cup). The more I found out, the more I found it interesting; I just listened to him telling me his story.

The more Joseph shared, the more parallels I found

with my own story. I felt like finally, I'd found someone who understood.

Something I had often thought about and feared going into a new relationship, was having to share my story from the beginning, never knowing how honest to be, as mine is definitely a story that is still being written. For me, telling my story meant being vulnerable and trusting in another person, which Joseph made so much easier by being so open and honest with me straight away.

Joseph, at the age of twenty-two, after battling with addiction for a couple of years (and with the help of a family friend), found the rooms and started going to meetings. Here he found a sponsor and started his personal journey through the 12-step programme. The more I have come to learn about his own story, which like mine is still being written, the more I fall in love with Joseph. He has shown me a courage and determination most people never find, because simply they are too scared to start looking.

Within the first week of us knowing each other, I told Joseph everything, and he made me feel safe, and calm, two feelings I never thought I would have used to describe my life, and all because I knew he would get it. Our struggles weren't too dissimilar and when he said he understood, I believed him. I could tell by the questions he asked. Then, just a week later, we met in person for the first time.

I'd just finished another dinner with my mum one evening and had lied to her (at the age of twenty-seven), telling her that I needed to leave early to be there for a friend, bearing in mind it was peak lockdown at the time. Instead, I went to meet Joseph on a bench, by the Thames path in Canary Wharf.

Apprehension quickly faded and I felt excited when I saw him approach me. In his presence, I was instantly at ease. Looking out across the city of London, Joseph and I sat and talked like we'd done it forever. That bench will forever have a very special memory for us!

I still think about the fact that I was never meant to move to Canary Wharf. If COVID hadn't delayed things for me, or if we had met a couple months earlier when I was still in the thick of it, I would never have met Joseph.

A couple of months later my visa for Singapore was finally granted, but suddenly I had reason to stay.

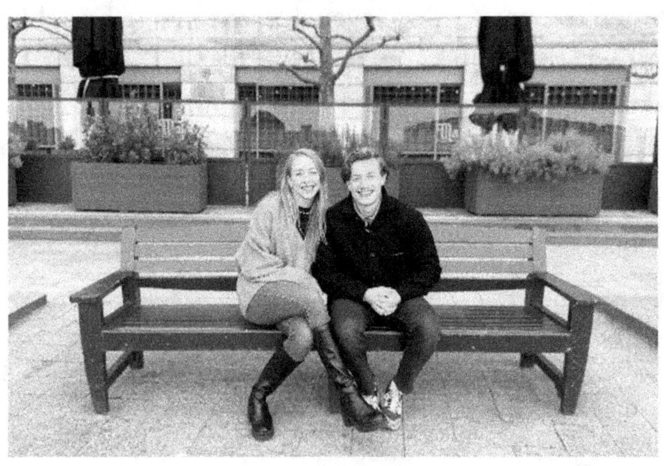

The famous bench, on our two-year anniversary 29.01.23

Chapter Ten

TWENTY-NINE

'It can be very beneficial to get involved and take action in the field of mental health and eating disorder awareness and prevention.'

As I turned tewnty-nine, the world felt very different to me. I felt calm where there had been so much noise, for so much of my life.

Now I know what I went through does not define me and is not my whole story. It has, however, forced me to really look at myself and learn why I did the things I did and why I felt certain things. I know that some of my behaviours could be generations of similar behaviours being passed on throughout communities and within families and they could also be the result of minute moments of learning from my childhood, which were incorrectly interpreted and held onto. I am still learning.

Beyond what has been written, my full story will continue to evolve, which I think is a beautiful thing about life; we can always (if we want to), keep growing.

What I am confident about now, is that the way I view myself is different. I am kinder to my inner child, and the way I process emotion, is rational and raw. Now, where I need to, I ask for help, always. I am not ashamed to speak out or admit when I am suffering, because I've found that success is about having the right people and mechanisms around you to be able to cope, and now that my relationship with food is healthier, more balanced and intuitive, I can cope. I am not saying I never have bad days, of course I do, I just recognise them and face them with the full force of my new education and my inherent determination.

Eventually, Mum left to return to Malaysia and my relationship with Joseph continued. She had met Joseph, and she knew that I was being left in good hands. He inspired me to work on my recovery, as I saw him work so hard for his own.

I have come to realise that Joseph's story has a definite crossover with mine. For so long, especially in the recent years of my recovery, people close to me had listened, but I always felt like they never really got it. Joseph did.

Before Joseph, I hadn't considered myself to have had an addictive personality and did not really understand what it fully meant. I was just disciplined, or at worst a bit too competitive. The difference today is I am able to recognise, understand and accept myself for all my flaws including this, which allows me to have a healthy and manageable balance in my life.

You might've heard the phrase 'control the controllables', which is only possible when you understand what is truly in your control. It took me time to see this, but I try to remember it in every situation I am in, and for every adversity I face.

These days, Joseph and I both focus our energy into the gym and our fitness-focused lifestyles. Others might still see this as obsessive, but we both enjoy it (it's part of who we are) and we know how important it is for us to help manage other aspects of our life. We chose to spend our time this way and it brings us so many other benefits. Besides, doesn't it say more about society that we continue to question when someone spends hours a day in a gym or does not drink alcohol, yet we don't think twice when someone sits in front of a TV for hours or in a pub garden having beers?

We've been together for over two years now, moving in together after six months and still we get closer every day. Joseph understood me from the beginning and continues today to make me want to be the best version of myself. Wonderfully, we have supported each other's growth through recovery, and will continue to grow as time goes on. Ultimately, we see each other's potential for the future, and we truly want to face it all together. More than anything, Joseph keeps me grounded and with him I feel an overwhelming sense of calm.

Joseph has spent the last four years (since he first decided to become sober), creating a life with peaceful intentions and I am so grateful he shares that with me: *When you know, you know.*

I know that I am lucky, but by no means am I saying that a relationship or person will be the answer for everyone struggling. Joseph and I both worked hard on ourselves, to understand who we really were, and timing is everything. When we met, we were sure of ourselves and our paths to recovery and not willing to compromise certain daily behaviours that were crucial to keeping my bulimia and his sobriety under control. The potential of our relationship working was never going to put our recovery in jeopardy; we both knew it was not worth risking our own recovery.

Separately, and before we knew of each other, we each took the time, the painful time and the periods of uncertainty to make real changes for a brighter future, for ourselves. We both recognised that the path would not always be clear for us and that things might get really tough, but with hope we built ourselves back up and now, today, we get to share that life together. I'm lucky, because for us, it did work, and we found that together we really are stronger.

Of course, there are days that are harder, and I might struggle to communicate but I trust Joseph to ask, *"Are you ok?"*

Now I am more aware, I am able to look outward and see just how prevalent disordered eating is. Too many of my friends have experienced some of the same struggles, at the same time I did and sadly I think one of them continues to suffer today.

Back then, life felt so lonely, I was sure I was in this alone, but now, I reflect on the fact that most of my friends had very similar thought patterns and worries – if only we knew or had the courage to speak to each other!

Today, lots of people are aware of eating disorders, or disordered eating behaviours, yet there is still a lot of stigmas attached and preconceived judgments around what it all means. There are generational differences too, in the interpretation of eating disorders and what causes them, and this further contributes to why so many are still suffering. Adding in things like social media and the way society functions today, I really do think there is a huge misunderstanding in the way we approach recovery and in helping those suffering with understanding their own illness.

I'm proud of the person I am today, of the woman I've grown into and proud of the way I've overcome some big internal battles. I've learned a lot from what I've been through and while I hope no one ever experiences the desperation and darkness as I did, especially at such a young age, there is no doubt that I wouldn't be the person I am today without my bulimia.

Understandably, I regret the fact that I lost over eight years of my life to this illness, and the ripple effect this had on my relationships with those closest to me, but that's my only regret. I don't blame myself for my actions. I don't blame anything or anyone for my actions, no one intended for this to happen to me, least of all me!

I continue, to this day, to work hard to understand the *why* and to uncover the underlying factors that led me to suffer with bulimia for as long as I did. Part of this process has been to share my story in the hope that it might save others all that unnecessary time wasting and suffering and help them on their recovery journey sooner.

One of the biggest things I've learned is, this was no one's fault. But I also now know that it does not need to be like this. Through direct support, better understanding, and more open conversation, I really believe we can help hundreds of thousands of people more!

I have had to come to terms with how I treated so many people in my life, throughout the years that I was suffering, particularly my parents; I took out a lot of my anxieties on them. They loved me the most and I treated them the worst. Now, I know that my younger self was in too much pain to know any better, if only I could have just vocalised and asked for help before my bulimia spiralled the way it did ...

I also know it was never an intention of mine to push away and hurt the people I love most (it was purely a defence mechanism), and now I strive all the time to make up for that lost time and those missed chances. Thankfully, I always knew deep down they loved me unconditionally and supported me as best they could. And now, having had the chance to discuss everything in detail and create a safe space for the vulnerable conversations, my parents understand so much more and our relationship is stronger than ever.

It's important to me that people see the bigger picture in my story. I am not a victim, I'm just a person who didn't know where to turn as a child, a child who through lack of understanding internalised all of their pain but found their way in the end. I am not saying I have all the answers, and the ending is not perfect, but today, I am better than I was yesterday and tomorrow I will be better than I am today. That's what it's all about. And now, I want to raise awareness of the issues that plagued me and that must start with a focus on childhood and where certain beliefs and rules may have stemmed from. Maybe it was one comment from a stranger? Or a piece of clothing that did not fit? I know there will always be potential triggers in our lives, but what's most important is how we learn and choose to cope. That's where the difference is.

In writing this book, I want people to see there's another way. If I had had an honest story to relate to, back when I was twelve, I know I wouldn't have felt such loneliness or maybe I would have had more courage to tell someone and so I'm hoping with my book, someone else can feel that too. The earlier we can start having these conversations the more impact they will have, and the less suffering will occur.

Everything I did during those eight years, seems so shocking for a young girl to go through, but I can guarantee I'm not the only one and sadly, I'm very aware that I won't be the last. Now, I feel driven to raise awareness and to normalise talking about this, without anger, frustration, and shame.

To do this, it's important that we reframe the

conversations around disordered eating. We need to recognise that these young people are acting out and help them to realise that it's likely not even about body image and is more about avoiding uncomfortable, likely new, emotions. It's just that sometimes, our bodies feel like the only things in our control.

Being with someone in recovery has allowed me even more insight into the way our minds work, and I've witnessed the bravery in people sharing their stories. I think, if schools had platforms of a similar nature, ones that encouraged sharing and reflection, (perhaps anonymously for children), we could see an incredible impact on young people's confidence and resilience – *a problem shared is a problem halved!*

In today's culture of social media dominance, we can't forget to question the uses of filters and photoshop when we see glamorous photographs on social media; doing so will put things into perspective. These photos are just a highlight reel, a manipulation of real life, which is easy for me to say now – so rational and logical. But imagine a child thinking like that? Even I need reminding and dedicated time away from the platforms, otherwise the cost of comparison is too much on my mental health. That's why we need constant intervention to point out the body image parameters that society has created, are false and do not make us feel fulfilled, happy, and content.

We need to educate and raise children to feel safe to share their emotional vulnerabilities as this will help prevent internalised trauma and provide the biggest opportunity for growth. They need to know that not every emotion will be easy to understand, but we need to give them the opportunity to go through that in a safe space where they feel like they can vocalise their feelings and ask for help when they need it. I hope to have inspired this with my own story and the extremities I experienced so that those who can relate, have a chance to. Even if it means friends or parents have a better idea of what questions to ask.

When it comes to food, we need to educate our children about macronutrients and the effects nutrients, or the lack of them, can have on their growing bodies. We should do this while also examining our language around food and commit to not associating the words 'good' or 'bad' with them. In turn, our children can educate their children and break that desperate cycle of controlling, harmful behaviours linked to associating our worth with how we physically look. So many conversations around food are associated to how we feel emotionally and our appearance, when in reality the only link should be a scientific one, the fuel that our body requires to take on the physical demands of the day.

A final note from me ...

I have a tattoo on my back taken from the quote, below, which I chose as an expression of my commitment to my recovery. Looking back on my twelve-year-old self, desperately striving for a perfection that was impossible to achieve (because, in my mind, I kept changing the goalposts and was never good enough), I am reminded of both how far I've come and of how I still have far to go.

"Accept that you are imperfect and always will be. Your quest is not to perfect yourself, but to better your imperfect self." Eric Greitens

For years I was looking to be fixed, when actually, I needed to accept that I would carry this for the rest of my life, and that it's OK. It was my perception and my mindset towards myself that needed to change. What I do with it and how I chose to react and learn from my journey with my bulimia is what defines me, not the illness itself. No one is perfect, and everyone has a story, so many people are afraid to read the pages because they fear what they might find. I have used my suffering to find meaning and a new sense of purpose and importance going forward, to try and make sense of my journey. Here is your chance and your encouragement to make the most of yours.

Jade.

FROM THE OUTSIDE

As an adult, I'm very aware of the important role we play in the shaping of young minds, but I can't tell you what it was like to be around those that suffer as I was lost in my own turmoil. I'm so grateful that my parents have agreed to contribute to my book from their own perspective, which we hope will provide a small glimpse of the struggle they faced and add to the conversation.

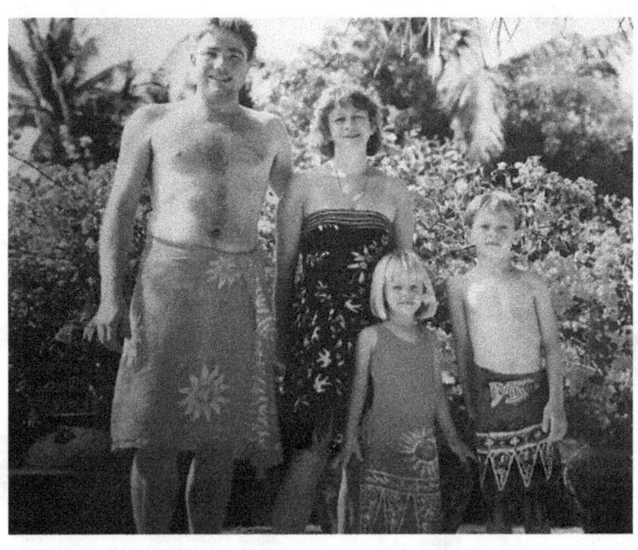

Family photo in Bali, one of my favourites

A father's perspective ...

Jade was always a difficult eater, at least compared to her brother, who ate basically everything and had a voracious appetite even from a very early age. He was experimental, either out of curiosity or a desire to please us, his parents, so he would happily order roti canai with a spoonful of laksa sauce on the top, while Jade would invariably stick to rice and egg ... it was safe and she would order it for every meal, especially when we were on holiday. I don't think she got any pleasure out of food, she ate out of necessity, rather than enjoyment.

So by the age of seven she decided to stop eating meat and only occasionally ate seafood, and by nine that went as well and she became a vegetarian, which as principal cook in the house was quite irritating as I had to cook two meals most days, but we accepted it, if only as a compromise for her to eat more.

Warning bells should have started ringing then, but like most habits, we just accepted it. Whenever we went out as a family, Jade would pick at her food and only the promise of a Baskin Robbins, or similar, at the end of the meal would entice her to make a show of eating.

Jade was never fat, certainly not compared to western girls of the same age, but we lived in Asia and the smaller Chinese and Malay girls in her peer group looked malnourished by comparison.

However, in truth I was not aware of any major

underlying problem, and while we now know that from the age of twelve the situation got more serious, I certainly was blissfully ignorant, if anything her attitude to food was more exasperating to me than concern. She would come home from school and eat nutritionally rubbish cereal and biscuits and then claim she wasn't hungry when we sat down for our family dinner. For me family dinners were important, one place where we were all together and could discuss our respective day, I didn't really like the children to eat separately, as it was important family time, but always a little tense with Jade's restrictive eating habits and her brother teasing her reticence to try new things.

By fourteen, after much soul searching, and endless jungle walks with me, she chose to join her brother at boarding school in Singapore. He'd already been there for three years and was now in his final year and living in the senior boarding house, and hence was a cool brother to have there!

I was responsible workwise, for the Singapore office, so I would be down at least every other week for work and of course, prior to Jade arriving, would take Jade's brother out for dinner, which usually involved a lot of meat, restaurants like the Brazilian or Carnivore, just kept serving you the best cuts of meat till you called a halt. We both enjoyed this culinary extravaganza, as the food in the boarding house was basic to say the least and with a relatively large South Asian contingent, tended to be very dhal & rice based.

So, this changed when Jade arrived at UWC, although

they were only at the same school for one year, it was easier to take them out separately, with Jade to a vegetarian restaurant.

When her brother left for university, it was just vegetarian restaurants. I was not thrilled, but as Jade was never much fussed about eating, we would often just stay on the exec floor of the hotel I was staying in and eat snacks. We never ever talked about food! Jade had zero interest in expressing any interest in a restaurant or type of food at all.

Towards the end of her time in Singapore, one of her friends developed an eating disorder and lost so much weight over a relatively short time, that she was unrecognisable, this had never been the situation with Jade who mostly seemed to maintain her weight.

When she started purging, we put it down to alcohol or general unwellness, but it was her mum who first noticed this was becoming a habit. We saw a great example of this after her 16th or 17th birthday, where we had allowed her and her friends to have a room at the Park Royal hotel where we were also staying, so they all had somewhere to go after their night out.

The following morning the room looked totally trashed, there must have been ten seriously hungover girls in there in various states of disarray. Jade's mum had to sort out the room and eject her friends before we started the long drive back home to Kuala Lumpur. Unfortunately, it was a Saturday morning, so it seemed like half of Singapore were trying to get across the border into Malaysia to buy their weekly groceries. We were stuck on the border for hours, which gave Jade the opportunity to get out of the car and vomit several times.

But boarding school ended up being Jade's ally, she was off our radar most of the time, only holidays were an issue for her. And not unsurprisingly, Jade wanted to spend a lot of time on her own, only much later did we know why.

Two significant holidays come to mind, our once in a lifetime safari to South Africa, Zambia, and Botswana, this was meant to be the final big family holiday before her brother went to college, so Jade would have been sixteen. Looking back at the pictures, she looked dreadfully thin, but once again I'd been mentally putting this down to the second-rate boarding school food. Now, the food on this holiday was probably the best we'd ever had, and yet as usual Jade picked at it in a disinterested way and was generally a moody teenager, arguing with us and her brother the whole trip.

A few years later we went to Italy, for us an eating and sightseeing holiday, but this time Jade really got to me, her attitude to food was becoming not just tiresome but infuriating. Her mother was trying to be supportive, but even her patience was wearing thin and unfortunately, angry words were exchanged!

Looking back, Jade was really quite devious with her bingeing and purging. In 2011, I took her on a university look-see, after she had competed in the Touch Rugby World Cup in Edinburgh Scotland, representing Singapore. I had been at the grounds to see her play on each day, but she was always reluctant to have dinner with me afterwards.

On the final day, she went out with her team to party, and I was meant to pick her up from Glasgow train station at lunchtime. When I did, she looked a mess, but we stayed the night somewhere near Manchester, and I was looking forward to some quality time with her.

Unsurprisingly at this point, she didn't really want anything much to eat and certainly didn't want to drink anything, which under the circumstances was wise, but later when we went to our room she claimed she could not sleep and wanted to call her friends, so she disappeared for an hour or so ... this habit was repeated when we got to Nottingham and even when we stayed a night with friends in Saul ... constantly making excuses to 'disappear' for an hour or so ... I must have been really stupid not to notice a pattern here.

Although my attitude to this has changed significantly over the years, my feelings at the time were non-woke, which in hindsight I regret, but I was someone who had dismissed counselling as 'not for me'. At the time, yes, we knew she had some ill-defined eating disorder issues, but I remember thinking; don't most girls go through this?

Now, I better understand the trauma and anguish Jade has been under and the effect it has had on her physically and emotionally, but how do you prevent this for others going through the same life experiences? There will always be the media portraying an unrealistic avatar of what is expected of today's youth; didn't it start back in the sixties with Twiggy? How does one isolate us from this social conditioning?

So now we come to the bombshell letter Jade wrote to us ... were we surprised? Yes. Hurt? Of course, and remorseful that we could not have done more. From my point of view, while upsetting in the context it was written, it was good to get it into the open so we could discuss this; Jade has always preferred writing her thoughts and feelings, as opposed to verbalising them.

We are from different generations, mine just got on with things. In my day, we didn't have access to counsellors, or therapists, and maybe our lives would have been different if we had? I doubt it, but for Jade the counselling worked and now she has come out the other side with a desire to help others with a similar mental illness, for which, I salute her.

A mother's perspective ...

Jade was born in Malaysia and attended a local nursery, just up the road from our home; she called it the dinosaur school because of the big painting on the building. Jade loved it there and went on to enjoy school too, picking up good grades and having friendship groups. She was always sporty and competitive (like her dad), and always in awe of her brother, missing him when he went away to school.

Jade wasn't into traditionally girly dolls and playthings, instead she had a thing for soft toys and dressing up! She had always loved music from a young age too; it would settle her like nothing else.

As a young child she was so active. She'd enter the Junior Hash run and go tearing through the jungle each year, following a paper trail, playing in the waterfall and getting dirty. We would also go camping often, for weekends and she'd spend hours playing on the beach. Life was good.

At school, Jade always did well, and this continued when she went to boarding school to study for her Baccalaureate and IGCSEs. By this time, I knew there were issues for Jade around food and mealtimes, so I asked the houseparent of her dorm to keep a watchful eye on her, which I think she did, because Jade has since told me how overbearing she could be!

From a young age, Jade was never really interested in food, though we were a foodie family. And, when she first wanted to become a vegetarian, we decided this would only be realistic, if she actually enjoyed her vegetables that would sustain her bodies nutritional needs. Looking back at photographs, it's obvious she had a problem, but living with her at the time made it so hard to see the extent of the weight loss.

When I first became aware of her eating disorders, I tried to find a counsellor in Malaysia, but they were not specific to her age-related needs. As Jade was adamant that she was OK, I decided to try to manage her issues within the family. I've since found out that even though the dentist noticed the damage to her teeth, I wasn't made aware at the time there was a problem. Essentially, she was so secretive, that it made doing anything for her really hard. I tried to encourage her to talk each Sunday, when I asked her to get on the scales at home, so I could check she hadn't lost too much weight, but she'd become angry and wouldn't talk.

After her IGCSEs Jade went to Loughborough uni, (her brother was already at uni in the UK), and I stayed with her for a little while to help her settle. Afterwards, we spoke on the phone every day and we would come to our flat in Cheltenham to spend the summers with both children. While at university, Jade was active in all her sports and appeared to maintain her weight, so wrongly I assumed she was stable and coping well with her university life.

After that, we received Jade's letter out of the blue. We hadn't known things were that bad for Jade and we cried a great deal. We also thanked Jade for helping us to better understand her, but neither of us could comprehend how she'd coped and hidden things for so long; we talked a lot about that letter. Eventually, we found a world-renowned eating disorder specialist for Jade, in Cheltenham, and she worked hard seeing her once or twice a week.

If I could give advice to anybody else in my position, as the parent of a young person with bulimia, or any other disordered eating, it would be to never give up on them, no matter how hard they withdraw from you. I also think we need to examine our own behaviours. I remember going out to buy a dress for a wedding and feeling terrible, and saying out loud how I couldn't wear that because I looked so fat!

Ultimately, I have to admire Jade's strength and determination, she continued to play sport at national level, while battling an eating disorder.

These days, life is amazing; Jade is amazing! We talk most days and I feel so grateful for her – she's a joy to have in my life.

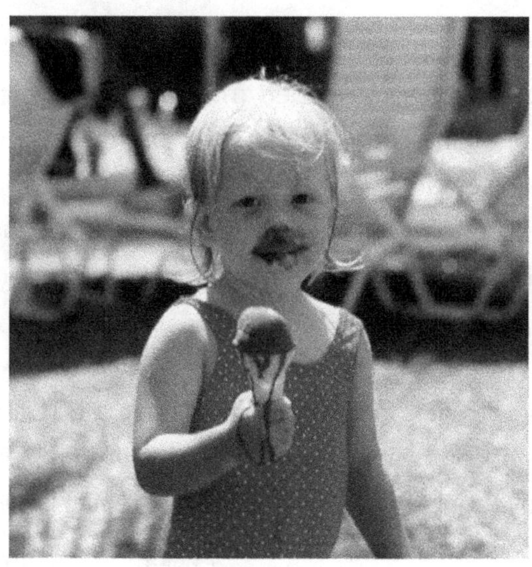

THOUGHTS ...

Preface: I appreciate the experience of disordered eating is different for everyone. The list below is from my experience and how I have chosen to interpret my disorder. I am not a medical professional, but I do believe the more we talk about our own stories, the more people will see their own similarities and differences and develop the courage to speak out and seek the help they need and deserve.

I was born as a unique individual into a world full of love and beauty. I was also blinded from my reality for far too long a time, by internal demons that told me how I should look, think, feel, and be. I lied, hid my true self, damaged relationships and, without knowing, abused my poor body over and over again. But slowly I learned, and I grew and now, I can fly.

I want to help others and cannot understate the usefulness of counselling therapy, especially when exploring disordered eating with someone who really knows their stuff. But I also know that the thought of it can be daunting.

From my counselling sessions, I took away some valuable tools:

- Breakdown the behaviours, one by one and try to uncover why you are choosing to restrict/binge/purge – can you see that you are ultimately using food as a form of control?

- There is always more to it that you might think, so don't stop exploring and settle on one revelation.

- Don't be afraid to share your story, even if it's a chat with a friend, or writing your story, just like I did mine. You never know who else might be suffering as its never obvious from the outside looking in.

- Ask for help, as directly as you are able to and don't stop until you find someone who can help in a way that is meaningful for you.

As happy as I am now, my heart will always contain a little sadness for the child I lost sight of. But what overrides this is that my heart is full of hope because now I am in control of my bulimia; it no longer defines me.

RESOURCES AND HELP LINES

(Unsurprisingly the resource and information available online is unhelpful and limited).

My personal details: jadegrantham.16@gmail.com
Instagram handle: jadegrantham1

BEAT Eating Disorders (UK)

- www.beateatingdisorders.org.uk/resource-index-page/
- www.beateatingdisorders.org.uk/get-information-and-support/get-help-for-myself/i-need-support-now/helplines/
- Email support for England: 0808 801 0677 help@beateatingdisorders.org.uk
- Email support for Scotland: 0808 801 0432 Scotlandhelp@beateatingdisorders.org.uk

- Email support for Wales: 0808 801 0433 Waleshelp@beateatingdisorders.org.uk
- Email support for Northern Ireland: 0808 801 0434 NIhelp@beateatingdisorders.org.uk

70 Resources to Support Eating Disorder Recovery

- www.onlinemswprograms.com/resources/resources-eating-disorder-recovery/

NHS – Advice for Parents

- www.nhs.uk/mental-health/feelings-symptoms-behaviours/behaviours/eating-disorders/advice-for-parents/
- www.nelft.nhs.uk/eating-disorder-resources

Some websites offer information in support of the friends and family of eating disorder sufferers

- www.mind.org.uk/information-support/types-of-mental-health-problems/eating-problems/for-friends-family/
- www.nationaleatingdisorders.org/learn/help/caregivers
- www.helpguide.org/articles/eating-disorders/helping-someone-with-an-eating-disorder.htm

REFERENCES

Prevalence of eating disorders by age, World, 1990 to 2019 - accessed 30.11.2022

Understanding The Rise of Eating Disorders in the UK - 2022 - accessed 30.11.2022

https://healthtalk.org/eating-disorders/secrecy-and-eating-disorders - accessed 05.12.2022

Lally, (2009) https://psychcentral.com/blog/need-to-form-a-new-habit-66-days - accessed 05.12.2022

https://www.nhs.uk/conditions/baby/weaning-and-feeding/babys-first-solid-foods/ - accessed 16.01.2023

Large et al (2019), https://medicalxpress.com/news/2019-01-people-susceptible-social-age.html - accessed 18.02.2023

The Impact of Acute Stress on the Neural Processing of Food Cues in Bulimia Nervosa (PDF, 150KB) https://www.apa.org/news/press/releases/2017/07/stress-brains - accessed 10.03.2023

Psychology Today, Carrie Gottlieb, PhD https://centerforchange.com/eating-disorders-and-romantic-relationships-how-to-cope-when-your-partner-has-an-eating-disorder/ - accessed 01.04.2023

https://www.verywellmind.com/coping-with-relapses-in-bulimia-recovery-1138291 - accessed 04.04.2023

Dr Agnes Ayton, the chair of the Eating Disorder Faculty at the Royal College of Psychiatrist, https://www.theguardian.com/society/2021/feb/11/doctors-warn-of-tsunami-of-pandemic-eating-disorders - accessed 04.04.2023

National Eating Disorders.Org https://www.nationaleatingdisorders.org/stages-recovery - accessed 04.04.2023

Lemoine, P. (2014, February 25). Giving Back in Eating Disorder Recovery, HealthyPlace https://www.healthyplace.com/blogs/survivinged/2014/02/giving-back-in-eating-disorder-recovery - accessed 11.04.2023

www.ingramcontent.com/pod-product-compliance
Lightning Source LLC
Chambersburg PA
CBHW062101270326
41931CB00013B/3166
* 9 7 8 1 3 9 9 9 7 4 8 0 6 *